Praise for YOUR Wor

"With the authenticity, humor, wisdom, and love of a good friend, Amy Connell invites readers to a right relationship with our bodies—a relationship grounded in our inherent worthiness as God's good creation. *Your Worthy Body* is a timeless invitation to grace and health, one that will outlast diets, fads, and trends because it is grounded in eternal truths. I am grateful for Amy's courage and willingness to pen this countercultural and necessary text for women of all ages and ethnic backgrounds who have struggled with body image (raises both of my cocoa brown hands) as we live into the balanced, free, and grace-filled lives promised by Jesus Christ."

—Rev. Donna Owusu-Ansah, author of *Loves...Regardless: Forty Devotions Inspired by Womanist Creative Thought and Theology*

"Women, even Christian women, have been bound up in a fabricated set of rules about fitness and diet for way too long. It's a type of bondage most have accepted as a joy-less life sentence. Amy Connell shines the truth and light in scripture so that women can be set free to embrace a life that is not just healthy but joy-filled!"

—Heather Creekmore, podcast host and author of *Compared to Who?* and *The Burden of Better*

"The overwhelming reason people present in my office is that they don't truly understand their identity in Christ and just how very loved and accepted they are, just as they are. They go on diets, wear the latest fashion, cook Pinterest worthy meals and yet still feel inadequate. *Your Worthy Body* takes a deep dive into what God has to say about us and our bodies and dispels many of the myths we've mistakenly believed in our search for adequacy and sufficiency. Amy Connell helps us identify the lies that have taken us captive, and counters them not with the world's wisdom but with God's truth as we seek to learn more about how God perceives us."

—Dr. Michelle Bengtson, board certified clinical neuropsychologist, podcast host, and award-winning author of *Breaking Anxiety's Grip: How to Reclaim the Peace God Promises*

"Your body is most certainly worthy...a short statement that is as profound as it is compact. Wellness is a journey, and often we set off on that journey without three essential components; balance, grace, and freedom. Dogmatic following of established "rules" have left so many far from their goals and dreams. Amy is a rule-breaker who has found tranquility at the intersection of spiritual, physical, and mental health. Your Worthy Body is an incredible composition through Amy's rule-breaking wellness journey that will leave you full of grace, hope, faith, and health."

—Dr. Richard Harris, MD, PharmD, MBA,
host of *Strive for Great Health* Podcast

"The definition of fitness relates to ability, work capacity and physical performance but all too often the term fitness is mistakenly used to describe an individual's appearance. Many people struggle to maintain a physical appearance created by popular media images and overlook the fact that the true intent of exercise is to help the body achieve an optimal level of performance and health. It's important to remember that form follows function; if exercise is used to help the body perform better, then naturally the appearance will change.

In her book, *Your Worthy Body*, author Amy Connell does a brilliant job of shattering the fallacy of exercising for appearance and provides an insightful, practical and scientifically valid guide for the real purpose of exercise: to achieve optimal health in the body provided by your Creator. This book will help you to create a rewarding relationship with exercise and teach you how to use it to enhance your quality of life."

—Pete McCall, Fitness Educator, Author of *Ageless Intensity
and Smarter Workouts*, host of *All About Fitness* Podcast

"Amy artfully meshes sound nutritional science, human physiology, and a whole lot of grace, into this book. *Your Worthy Body* will give you the tools (and permission!) to break the rules that diet culture has set out before us and help you cultivate a more accurate view of holistic wellness in order to take health promoting actions that serve you and your body well."

Brittany Braswell, MS RDN, LD

YOUR Worthy Body

Find Freedom in Health by Breaking All the Rules

Be full of grace!

—Aylon

Paperback ISBN: 978-1-7377076-1-5

E-book ISBN: 978-1-7377076-2-2

Cover design by Steve Kuhn

Interior design by Rebecca Sutton

Photo by Lis Purdy

*I am not a doctor, physical therapist, or registered dietician.
The content provided herein is simply for educational purposes and
does not take the place of medical advice from your provider. Every
effort has been made to ensure that the content provided in this book
is accurate and helpful for my readers at the time of publication.
However, this is not an exhaustive treatment of the subjects. No liability
is assumed for losses or damages due to the information provided. You
are responsible for your own choices, actions, and results. You should
consult your personal medical professional for specific problems.*

To my husband.

Without your love, support, patience, grace, and always telling me I'm sexy, this book never would have happened.

Contents

PART THREE: COOL DOWN

INTRODUCTION

Does this scenario sound familiar?

I spent much of my formative years comparing my body to someone else's. And by the word "formative," I mean until about ten years ago. Whether it was overhearing another teen girl discussing her size or assessing the bodies in the group fitness mirror, I developed the habit for running an almost constant unconscious analysis of my size compared to someone else's. And that habit began with a familiar scene...magazine cutouts on a mirror.

The bathroom mirror of my high school years held a cutout of a swimsuit model "for inspiration." Just like I couldn't transform my green eyes to her chestnut hue, I couldn't achieve her hourglass figure either.

Don't get me wrong; I tried. I pulled out VHS tapes and felt the burn with chipper women who used copious amounts of hair spray. I jumped on the scale in the middle of the exercise tape to see if I'd lost weight yet and for some reason was always surprised and disappointed when I hadn't.

As I got older, the picture for inspiration was removed, but the goal remained taped in my mind.

I spent the better part of my twenties wanting the kind of abs that go well with a belly-button ring. I kept waiting and working for those abs before pulling the piercing trigger. It never happened.

After popping out two babies in twenty months, I spent my early thirties trying to be a hot mom. My husband told me (and still tells me) I was both a hot mom and a sexy wife, but I didn't believe it.

As my littles grew, my time became more flexible. I filled that space with teaching fitness classes, running, and anything else to work off the calories I shamefully ingested. Perfect eating and my imperfect body occupied more space in my brain than I care to admit.

Maybe you have felt the same conflict too. I'm sure your story isn't the same, but between the inspirational cutouts, obsessive weight checks, and guilt-ridden eating, perhaps you feel something echo within your own life. If so, you're in the right place.

While I was investing my time growing as a fitness professional, I began doing the same for my spirituality by devoting more time with God. My weekly Bible studies intensified my faith, my church provided lessons in growing my relationship with Jesus, and my morning quiet time with Him became more sacred.

In hindsight, I think that was God teeing me up to hear His gentle whisper: *You're spending more time thinking about the food you're going to eat and the exercise you're going to do than you are about me.*

I wish I could say I immediately dropped my obsession with eating perfectly and having a #fitspiration body. Instead, that whisper planted a mustard-sized seed. It took time, but eventually, that seed took root and began growing into something new. God was giving me a new way to live a healthy life but without shame and self-loathing. The words of Isaiah come to mind:

> *See, I am doing a new thing! Now it springs up; do you not perceive it? I am making a way in the wilderness and streams in the wasteland.*
>
> Isaiah 43:19

God gave me a new focus. He took me from wandering the wilderness of perfection to greener pastures of grace. He's given this to me in my personal and professional fitness path.

My career as a fitness professional began as a new mom who wanted to create a program to work out with my baby. That baby is sixteen now. Just like he's grown from a twenty-inch bubbly baby to a six-foot-two witty young man, my teaching and training philosophy has changed.

Early on, much of my energy aimed at following all the health rules I read about and saw on the morning shows. I foolishly assumed my clients desired the same. I sensed something different from my older clients, though I could never put my finger on it. Now that I'd be considered an "older client," I get it.

Health isn't just about looking a certain way. It's not a list of dos and don'ts. It's not a static adjective...hot, fit, perfect. It's a verb. It's a fluid behavior and attitude. My ideal health has changed as I've aged; I bet yours has too. I liken the word "health" to the Greek word *agape*, or "love" in the Bible. *Agape* love is unconcerned with the self and concerned with the greatest good of another.[1]

What if we swapped the words "*agape* love" for health in that definition? *Health is unconcerned with the self and concerned with the greatest good of another.* Our health is less concerned with how we look and more about being physically equipped to love others. This falls right in line with a sermon I heard that changed everything I understood about health: We take care of our bodies so we can do what we are called to do. We'll dig into this idea more in "Your Body Works for You."

Now, whether I'm training middle-school girls or empty-nester women, I'm acutely aware of my language and message. No longer do I market "New Year! New You!" (Because what is wrong with you in December?) I don't speak of the f-word (fat) or audibly lament the extra pounds I may be carrying.

Instead, I ask my clients to tune in to how they feel while exercising. I want them to notice the muscles they are working. My conversation with teen girls revolves around finding joy in their movement or exploring why we move the way we do. Most of my adult women are over forty. It's not unusual for them to work around cranky knees, creaky backs, or other complaining body parts. So do I. The exercises we do strengthen weak areas to prevent injury and promote mobility—not to lose a quick pound.

This new thing also gave me a new perspective on the health and fitness industry. Yes, the industry inspires and motivates others to move and eat well. Unfortunately, the ads, messaging, and even challenges create a side effect: shame.

Shame researcher and author Dr. Brené Brown defines shame as:

> *the intensely painful feeling or experience of believing that we are flawed and therefore unworthy of love and belonging—something we've experienced, done, or failed to do makes us unworthy of connection.* [2]

Somewhere along the way, the fitness industry has told us if we don't execute their rules perfectly, we aren't enough. Lose more weight. Lift more pounds. Run farther. Get your diet right. Eat this new plan; last year's was wrong.

But dig a few layers in, and you'll find it causes a fragile core (and I don't mean muscles) that relies on adherence to rules to tell us if what we are doing is enough.

We don't feel like we're doing enough when:

- We don't exercise for a full hour.
- Our daily food intake isn't perfectly executed.
- We miss a workout.
- We eat carbs—the horror!

These rules have overtaken our definition of success. When we see that morning-show segment or read the BuzzFeed article containing any superlative (best, most, or anything ending in -est), we file that in the "goals" category. Best is acceptable. Anything less is not.

Then, when our "best workout for weight loss" is cut short because our child wants to open up about an issue, or the "perfect weeknight meal" is a flop and we pull out a frozen pizza, we feel like a failure. Perhaps we even feel unworthy of our fitness, food, or body.

I'm here to stop the madness.

You are worthy. Your effort is worthy. Your body is most certainly worthy. And you don't need man-made rules to live out this truth.

I hope you see by now this isn't your typical health and fitness book.

Within each chapter of this book, I take a rule set forth by the health industry, social media, and perhaps even ourselves and rebuke or refine that rule with science and/or scripture. Each of these rules is part of my story and one I previously tried to keep. Do you need to break all of these rules as well? Not at all. But I do encourage you to take stock of what you hold true and why.

Most chapters have applicable resources. My dad taught me long ago to never present a problem without also providing a solution. In the upcoming pages, I'll provide a rule to break and some ways you can tweak that rule to make it work for you. Or, as in "Pass the Bucket," I'll give you recipes and tools to prevent the need for one. The end of this chapter holds a QR code that will take you directly to the online resource guide, where you can download or view everything in one place.

Whether or not you utilize the resources, I want to empower you to figure out what kind of moving and eating is best for *you*. As I said, this is not a manual or a quick-fix guide. Consider it a choose-your-own-adventure book in which you are in control of your next steps. And the best part of those books? If you don't like where you're heading, you can go back and change your path. You can do the same with this book.

In this book, you're given plenty of information and options to make the next right choice for you. And yes, you'll see that my story and perspective is presented through the lens of my faith, but no matter how (or if) faith is part of your story, there is room for you in these pages. You are welcome on this journey.

One more thing: This is not a book of my meandering daydreams. It's a culmination of nearly twenty years as a fitness professional and exercise science and nutrition geek. I feel like this is also the time to acknowledge that there are many fitness leaders and registered dietitians who have more letters and education after their names than me. Some of these leaders are mentioned throughout this book. I honor and respect their work. The research they provide enables me to bring you a condensed version of the countless studies and books they produce. While I may act like a know-it-all, in fact I do not know it all (also true in about every area of my life). But I keep learning and reading and gathering information to pass on to you.

Part of my learning process resulted in an unintended consequence: I am more gentle with myself. Yes, you read that correctly. I've become more gentle in my expectations, workouts, and body image. Most importantly, I've learned to give myself grace and enjoy the process rather than fixate on an unattainable goal. I want that for you too. It's glorious.

What I promise you'll receive from this book are balance, freedom, and grace. When you close this book for the final time, you will have science- and scripture-backed ways to find those. You'll be confident to move and fuel your body in a way that works for you and how God made you. You'll have plenty of resources nestled in most chapters to do this. And I pray...oh I pray that you have a renewed spirit and mind in your movement, nutrition, and body.

Ready? Let's dig into science and scripture to discover the grace and freedom God has for us. And yes, you can grab a little bit of chocolate for the trip.

As I mentioned, most chapters offer resources. All are included in these pages, but if you'd like one place to access the recipes, charts, tables, and multiple movement videos, scan the QR code below and receive them all in one location. Simple, huh? Speaking of simple, you'll also receive a "Simple Take" at the end of each chapter. Sometimes I feel overloaded with information and appreciate a summary of what was just presented. "The Simple Take" will ease that information overload by providing a simple summary of each chapter's main point.

PART ONE: WARM UP

When I was in my twenties, you could drop me in the middle of any group fitness class and I could join with ease. My heart ramped up quickly, and my muscles participated without complaint. I do not recommend this to anyone, by the way.

But twenty years later? Without priming my body properly, I'm almost guaranteed to injure myself. And if I'm lucky enough not to get hurt, I won't get as much out of the workout because I didn't enter into it prepared.

Just like our bodies need to warm up in order to get the most out of a workout, in this section, we are going to warm up our minds. Throughout this book, I'm asking you to think differently. Later I give you applicable ways of doing this in your movement and eating. But first, I want to prime the way we think about our body, how we define a healthy body, and why we even want a healthy body in the first place.

Cue the music. Let's start.

CHAPTER ONE

I'm supposed to look a certain way

Quick: Create a mental picture of what you think you're supposed to look like. Hold onto this image; we will come back to it.

Several years ago, I was at a local restaurant eating lunch. As I left, I spotted a friend with a group of ladies at a different table. I stopped to say hi, and my friend introduced me to the other women.

"This is Amy Connell. Oh! We were just talking about working out... Amy teaches fitness classes at the neighborhood multipurpose fields."

Then I saw it. We were exchanging pleasantries, but I caught that split-second flicker I've witnessed so many times. One of the women I was just introduced to scanned my body from the top of my head down to my knees and back up. She may not have even realized she did it, but I knew what it meant: *Is her body worthy of being a fitness professional?*

Maybe you've experienced that when you say you're headed to the gym. Or when you try a new nutrition plan. Or say you do anything health-wise. That quick once-over to establish credibility. Worthiness.

Unless you opened this book without reading the title, you can guess my response: Yes, your body is worthy.

What is it, exactly, that causes us to question the worthiness of how our body looks, moves, and fuels? (And if you don't question these things—yay! But also stick with me in this chapter. It's the starting point of our journey.)

I've read, listened, and wrestled with the complexities of health and body image for years. And I've come up with a few areas that prompt us to hold certain things to be true, question our worthiness, and provoke us to think we are supposed to look a particular way.

Stories from our youth

Think back to your younger years. This might be awkward middle-school years, angsty high school years, or advancing college years. What words did the people around you say about you and your body? Were you told you were unathletic? The "big one" of the family? Slow? Too short? Too tall? Words have power. The stories we heard about ourselves growing up impact how we see ourselves now. It may be that we are holding on to something that was never true.

I've always been self-conscious of my abs. For as long as I can remember, I've felt I have a flabby belly. I think it stems from an offhand comment somebody made years ago. It's the first thing I check out when trying on clothes, and it determines whether or not I like how an article of clothing fits me. A few years ago, I took advantage of a Groupon and booked a full-body scan that analyzed muscle, body fat, and bone density in each region of my body. Why? Quite simply, I was curious. Through this scan, I learned that my right leg has nearly a pound and a half more muscle than my left and my bones are very dense. I also learned that not only do I have low visceral (deep belly) fat, my abdomen is the leanest area of my body. Huh? You mean all this time I've been obsessed with my abs and they have the least amount of adipose (body fat)? I'd named myself as big-bellied and held on to that for way too long.

The words you've lived under may be a rickety shack of lies rather than a firm foundation of truth. If that's the case, it's time to release those and find some new, more life-giving words to live by. Words that are true, noble, right, pure, lovely, admirable, excellent, and praiseworthy (we'll talk more about this in Chapter 3).

Messaging from our American culture

As I write in 2021, our society values lean, sculpted bodies. Fifty years ago, women's curves were desired. And somewhere between the waiflike bodies on the television hit *Ally McBeal* and today, big juicy behinds became a *thing*.

The history of American beauty is nearly indefinable. Rumor has it American beauty Marilyn Monroe donned a size twelve in 1945 (which is purportedly comparable to a size six to eight today),[1] but what about other periods? What messages have women been told throughout American history?

Consider these time periods:

- 1920s: flat chest, downplayed waist, bobbed hair, boyish figure
- 1930s–1950s: curves, hourglass figure, large breasts, slim waist (pinup girls)
- 1960s: willowy, thin, long slim legs, adolescent physique
- 1980s: athletic, svelte but curvy, tall, with toned arms
- 1990s: waifish, extremely thin, translucent skin, androgynous
- 2000s to today: flat stomach, "healthy" skinny, tan, large breasts and butt, thigh gap[2]

As someone born in 1974, please explain how I can achieve all the standards outlined in my lifetime: having an extremely thin yet curvy body with large breasts while still appearing androgynous and still walking around with a thigh gap between my athletic legs and large butt? GAH!

The world is fickle. If we let it determine whether we feel good about how we look or not, we'll never keep up.

Thanks to social media (and I do mean this sincerely), we are starting to see all body shapes and sizes represented. I give credit to Dove Soap and their "Real Beauty" campaign for spearheading this effort in 2004. I witnessed different body shapes and colors represented at various retailers, which brings me so much joy (and my business to them). We are getting there, but unfortunately for every picture of a real-sized woman, it seems there's another filter added to Instagram to widen our eyes or create the illusion of six-pack abs.

As I've deepened my understanding of health, I've also realized my version of an ideal body is tightly constrained. Magazines and television shows of my youth portrayed thin white women. So did commercials and billboards. Between my age and my white skin, it never occurred to me that a thin body wasn't what everyone strived for. It turns out our culture of origin impacts what we think we are supposed to look like as well.

Expectations of our culture of origin

In 2003, my husband and I loaded a big-screen box TV, our nine-month-old's crib, and the rest of our belongings in a truck and moved to Houston, Texas. The area we now live in is one of the most diverse counties in the United States. I have truly cherished getting to know the different experiences of friends and neighbors. My suburban neighborhood is a menagerie of color and culture, and it delights me to no end.

Our country continues to grow in its diversity as well. As of 2020, 40 percent of America identifies as Hispanic, Black, Asian, Native American, Pacific Islander, or a combination of these. The other 60 percent have white European roots, though it's expected that by 2045, that number will have dropped to slightly less than 50 percent.[3]

We just discussed how the traditional American culture has influenced us, but have you considered that not all cultures have the same "body ideal?" Countless articles and books are written about cultural body image. I'm certainly no authority on this, but I have made the effort to glean from the wisdom of those who are experts. Those experts are women who have grown up with influences and expectations. I asked a Facebook group of women in my community, "Would you be willing to share what culture you identify with and what is traditionally considered beautiful, desirable, etc.?" As expected, the responses varied among cultures.

Consider the feedback provided by these ladies' personal experiences, noted here in their own words:

- *Vietnam*. "Traditionally Vietnamese women should be skinny with flawless, porcelain white skin with long straight black hair. Your skin color depicts your social status; dark skin means you work outside."

- *Nigeria*. "Ideally, our people like shapely women. Long legs, big butt, wide hips. Short women get made fun of. It doesn't really matter if you're skinny or fat, as long as you have a Coke-bottle shape. The shape of a person's nose is a huge deal for people in Eastern Nigeria. Overall, what Nigerians consider beautiful is very diverse compared to other countries in my opinion."

- *India*. "First on the list would definitely be fair skin. The other thing that really matters for Indians is beautiful eyes; we are obsessed with big eyes with beautiful lashes and eyebrows. Indians generally don't like skinny women...but not too heavy either. We also want a sharp pointed nose and medium to long hair."

- *China*. "There are three main components: hair (black, long, and rich), face (fair skin, shiny eyes, and a small mouth), and a body (slim but curved shape, often described as 'soft' to be considered good). Muscles or scars were undesirable by girls or women from noble or rich families because they were normally associated with lifestyles of farmers or workers."

- *African American*. "Today's society looks for light skin, long hair, and big butt. The waist has to be smaller than the hips and weight doesn't matter too much as long as it's not tinkering on obesity."

- *Latina*. "My version of what is expected of a Latina is a lean body with curves. We also desire long, thick wavy hair. We do have curves but not necessarily lean ones, thanks to our delicious food!"

Obviously, women have different experiences, and these may not represent others from the same culture. Nevertheless, it's important to acknowledge that however your culture defines beauty, chances are there's another culture that desires something different.

I also can't overlook our American friends who are a blend of more than one race. In fact, the US Census reports that the "Two or More Races" category is expected to be the fastest-growing category over the next several decades.[4] America continues to be the melting pot it prides itself on. And thanks to the various ways families come together, we now see various cultures of origin under one roof. As the T-shirt of one of my clients says, "Families don't have to match."

The examples above can, and do, hold volumes in research and literature. This isn't even the tip of the iceberg, but I hope it helps you see the full construct that can sink our confidence in our uniquely created bodies. Perhaps we need to broaden our perspective of the "perfect body" and instead remember they are all from our perfect Creator.

Lack of contentment

I've been highlighting my hair since the eighth grade. It started by trying to take off the brassiness of continual perms, and now it covers up gray. I'm constantly looking for a product to help with the bags under my eyes, and on top of that, I apply plenty of concealer to the dark circles. I enjoy trying new facial products. Every six months, I debate whether or not I want to inject paralyzing toxins between my eyes to soften the two lines. I haven't yet, but check back six months from now. I admit I want to appear fresh and youthful. Perhaps I'm a little discontent. But I'm not alone.

In fact, an entire industry capitalizes on our discontentment. According to the Global Wellness Institute,[5] the personal care, beauty, and anti-aging market is valued at over $1 trillion. That's trillion with a T. Healthy eating, nutrition, and weight loss is worth over

$700 billion, and the fitness and mind/body category is valued at almost $600 billion. That's over $2 trillion focused on changing our bodies and how they age.

Yes, there is some benefit to these industries. As a personal trainer and nutrition coach, I add to these numbers in the hopes of helping people develop healthy lifestyles. But my hope for my clients is not for them to achieve a certain size. It's to equip them to be able to do what they are called to do. In general, however, these industries prey on the discontentment we have from our graying roots down to what color our toenails are.

How I wish I could live out the words of the apostle Paul, who wrote:

> *For I have learned to be content in whatever the circumstances. I know what it is to be in need, and I know what it is to have plenty. I have learned the secret of being content in any and every situation, whether well fed or hungry, whether living in plenty or in want.*

Philippians 4:11–13

We may be discontent with our body because we haven't been taking care of it. That's fair. Or perhaps our bodies have experienced health issues that have caused significant changes.

But there's a spectrum between contentment and cultivating perfection. Contentment offers unconditional satisfaction. Cultivating perfection never satisfies...because what is perfect anyway? We may land closer to one side or the other. But my hope is these pages shift us closer to the satisfaction of knowing we are taking care of ourselves rather than taking care of how we look. Maybe we can inch our way to contentment rather than worrying so much about the inches around our hips.

The influence of other bodies

On Instagram, I follow several hashtags. One is #christianfitness. While I value different experiences and perspectives, I particularly like to see posts in the world of faith-based fitness.

May I be honest? Sometimes these posts are the opposite of encouraging. Why? Because often I see before and after pictures, with the "after" almost always demonstrating cut biceps, deltoids, and abs. The caption almost always gives a shout-out to God for the strength to do all things and a reminder that we are temples of the Holy Spirit.

I know the intent is to motivate and encourage. However, I *perceive* this: If I loved God enough, I'd have a better body. If I only relied on His strength more, I could look better in my gym clothes. I realize this is not the intention of these influencers. They love Jesus, I have no doubt. They do lean into Christ's strength. I do too. But the insecure fifteen-year-old hiding in me still finds herself comparing my body to theirs.

Comparison. In a heartbeat, I trade one verse for another. I shame myself for not having an Instagram-worthy temple but forget what the apostle Paul wrote to the Galatians:

> *Am I now trying to win the approval of human beings, or of God? Or am I trying to please people? If I were still trying to please people, I would not be a servant of Christ.*

> Galatians 1:10

Somewhere deep inside, I seek approval of humans and faces I only know through a screen rather than approval from God. This is not what God wants for me or why He gave me Jesus and His grace.

Make no mistake, our health is relevant. We need plaque-free arteries, a strong heart, and a clear mind. This is achieved through healthful living, which we will discuss even as we break the health rules throughout this book. But the basics of healthful living are this: Primarily eat the foods God gave us in their original state, and move our body in a way that brings us joy.

Doing these two things enables us to do what we are called to do. That may look like an inspiring Instagram picture. It may not. Your version of a healthy body is unique. Our body, our vessel, is to be prepared for anything He may call us to do. We honor God with our bodies by moving them and feeding them the foods He gave us. But never, not once, does He say it has to look a certain way.

Our inclination to follow the rules

If we've met over at my podcast, former blog, or anywhere on social media, you know me by my ministry name of Graced Health. This is the home base for everything I do in the health world. Grace isn't often associated with health. But it's critical to our overall well-being. It's not beating ourselves up over a missed workout or eating that dessert with your girlfriends. It's removing the running negative commentary in our brain. And it's allowing ourselves to not blindly follow the ever-changing health and fitness rules.

Jesus's time on earth consisted of demonstrating love in various forms to all people. He shook up the law...the rules...and taught that loving God and others was the foundation of everything. His brutal death and beautiful rising three days later extended forgiveness that previously had to be earned through acts and rituals. No longer did people have to follow the 613 rules outlined in the Old Testament. They just needed to follow Jesus Christ. His death and resurrection gave us grace for all the ways we mess up.

Perhaps it's time we give ourselves the grace Jesus died for. We do not have to hold ourselves to the 613 Old Testament rules that the Jewish people had to abide by. And we don't have to follow all the health rules either. A quick count on Wikipedia tells me there are 134 various diets people can follow.[6] Some of them are cringeworthy, by the way. While many are science-backed, I give others zero stars and do not recommend (feeding tube and cabbage diet: I'm looking at you).

We will break many health myths in this book, but it's not an all-encompassing list of rules. You may have seen additional ones that rub you the wrong way, or perhaps you've created your own. The point is to question what rules we feel like we need to follow, what we hold true, and why. Some rules may work for us; others will not. And I hope and pray we learn to give ourselves a lot of grace along the way.

Let's revisit that image you created at the beginning of this chapter. The one of what you think you are supposed to look like. Just like your unique makeup, it was formed through unique experiences, conversations, and expectations. My hope is that through this book, we take that vision and set it aside. We keep in mind the complexities that have formed that vision. We stop questioning why we don't look like we think we are supposed to and focus on meeting our body where it is. We find it worthy of movement, God-given foods, and most of all grace.

The Simple Take:
Despite what you may have seen, heard, and experienced, you do not need to look a certain way. Our unique bodies are evidence of the creativity of God, who never asks us to conform to a mold He didn't create.

CHAPTER TWO

Your body works for you

For years, when my friends would encourage me to start a blog, I scoffed. "The world does not need another health and fitness blogger," I'd respond. It didn't. The last thing the interweb needed was another white girl writing about recipes and easy ways to get movement in throughout your day (which, yes, I did both of these when I eventually did join the club). And, quite frankly, I had no interest in showing pictures of myself performing exercises while wearing only a sports bra and skimpy shorts. Besides, I didn't wear a sports bra and skimpy shorts, even in the privacy of my own home.

Eventually, though, the voices of my friends turned into whispers from the Holy Spirit. I'd like to tell you I immediately obeyed those soft callings. Nope. Instead, I responded in the most mature manner I could: I stuck my fingers in my ears, closed my eyes, and proclaimed, "I'm not listening!"

I'll let you figure out how that one turned out.

I spent the next several months figuring out all the intricacies of the writing world without posting anything. Then came the day I heard Mufasa's voice declare, "It is time." Yes, God spoke to me through James Earl Jones and the Disney classic *The Lion King*. I was finally ready.

Two days before the launch date, my family walked into our weekly church services. The series, "Not My Own," was designed to help our church family physically take care of themselves. I'm not proud of the thoughts I had as I walked into the building that day. I was there for worship and community. But the nutrition and fitness lesson? Snort. I exercised. I ate kale. I drink plenty of water. What was my pastor going to teach me that I didn't already know?

Oh sister, have you ever questioned God's messages? I believe my heavenly Father has a great sense of humor and relishes my earthly mind. I imagine a slight smirk as He looked at me and said, "Oh, you don't think you need this message? Try *this* on for size."

I didn't know then I needed the lesson of that sermon series: *We take care of our bodies so we can do what we are called to do.*

That statement rocked all I knew of health. You mean there's a connection? My body supports my faith? My body and my faith are intertwined? My body *doesn't* work for me and what I want it to do?

My faith had allowed me to become closer to my husband, to parent my children with more grace, and to step into volunteer roles to serve His marginalized children. But combining faith and health?

Mind-blowing.

I knew God had a purpose for me. I knew my current purpose was to write and share my story of searching for balance in an industry that screams extremes. My tagline was already established: balanced healthy living with a lot of grace and a little chocolate. I knew God wanted His daughters to find that balance and to stop beating themselves up over a missed workout or not perfectly executing their nutrition plan. In essence, He wanted them to break all these man-made rules and abide in His love and grace, regardless of how many servings of vegetables they had consumed that day.

That sermon's message took my focus away from how my body looked to how I used it to serve God. It gave language to what I had felt in my heart but didn't know how to articulate. Our bodies are created in all shapes and sizes, so it only makes sense that God simply asks us to take care of them to fulfill His unique plan for each of us.

What if, though, we have more than one calling? What if we have different kinds of callings that may or may not be impacted by a fast-food meal? And what, exactly, is a calling? How do we know what ours is? It's almost easier to think our body works for us rather than figure out how it's supposed to work for our calling.

If you're like me, those questions make you tense up your shoulders. We put so much pressure on the words "calling" and "purpose." Paul writes in Romans that *"we know God works for the good of those who love him, who have been called according to his purpose"* (8:28).

Merriam-Webster.com defines calling as a *"strong inner impulse toward a particular course of action especially when accompanied by conviction of divine influence."*[1] The Bible doesn't provide a definition, but considering the Ten Commandments and what we learn from Jesus, I believe it centers around using our God-given talents and gifts to glorify God and love and serve others.

Let's explore some of the ways God may be asking us to use our bodies to love and serve others.

Micro callings

Little daily callings. Moments and opportunities to love and serve others.

The day my son turned sixteen, I let him stay home from school to take his driver's test. (Because we all want to be cool moms sometimes, right?) Upon completion and passing (Yay! And ack!) I took him to a favorite brunch restaurant where he could order fried chicken and waffles. Yes, that's a thing in Texas. I can say I've never ordered this, though after asking for a bite to see what the hubbub was about, I affirm there's a reason for it being a thing.

He drove us home, which was quite fortuitous. I couldn't keep my eyes open. I didn't have the chicken and waffles, but I did order an omelet with cheese and a side of pancakes. Those pancakes were a fluffy, delectable mix of refined flour and sugar. The syrup exploded my taste buds as well as my blood sugar, only to crash later. Dairy and I don't get along. I know all this. We got home and I had a few precious hours with my firstborn before his friends got out of school and he drove off to see them. Unfortunately I didn't get to take advantage of that. All I could think of was *I. Must. Nap.* My body would not have it any other way.

That, my friend, is a micro calling gone wrong. The choices I made impacted my day. While it began as a special mother-son time, I lost the opportunity to fully capitalize on it. That nap prohibited spontaneous conversations and the simple enjoyment of my child. Had I not napped, my body still would have made it clear that it wasn't feeling its best. The brain fog set in and the energy waned. That time lost was not how I wanted the afternoon to look.

I experience micro callings in other ways: getting an afternoon project done, checking on a sick friend, and making sure I have enough energy to parent past 7:00 p.m. My podcast interviews are often held in the afternoon, and I know my brain needs to be clear and sharp. Micro callings don't have to be momentous occasions, but it's important I'm physically able to take each next step that God calls me to do.

Creative callings

Using the intricacies of how God made you to bless others and fill your own soul.

My former neighbor blessed neighbors and friends with parties and get-togethers. If you've ever read the book *Bread and Wine*, by Shauna Niequist, this is the kind of person who embodies joy around the table and nourishing one's friends. Not only is my friend amazing in the kitchen, but her home is also filled with gorgeous paintings created from her own hand and brush. In fact, if you ever visit my home, you'll see several of her creations.

We may not all be able to paint masterpieces. I certainly can't. But blessing others with our creativity can come in other ways. Maybe you scrapbook each year of your child's life for him or her to enjoy later. A couple of months into the COVID-19 pandemic, a friend doodled her representation of the times. She showed a world surrounded by masks, family units, playing cards, and first responders, all centered around the word "hope." When she shared it on Facebook, she blessed others by visually demonstrating the complexity of the season.

Spring 2020 also allowed seamstresses a time to shine. All of a sudden, the world was asked to wear a mask in public. Since most of us didn't have extra ones lying around (though I now I have about twelve), those who were comfortable with a sewing machine created masks for us to brave public domains. Speaking of sewing, my neighborhood Facebook group highlighted a woman who took neckties from a friend's late father and created a custom pillow from them.

Even picking a few flowers and strategically placing them in a vase can lift someone's spirits.

All of these acts show women who took their God-breathed gifts and blessed others in one way or another.

We certainly can't discount how sacred creativity is to God. If you doubt it, step outside and watch the sunrise (or set). Take notice of the colorful butterflies and birds. Peek outside an airplane window, and observe the landscape. His creative hand is evident in all of nature, just waiting to bless us. Look for inventive ways to bless others to experience this calling.

Servanthood callings

Supporting others with our gifts, talents, or presence.

One of the greatest adventures in the Old Testament is the book of Exodus, which recounts God's rescue of the Israelites from Egypt. God sent Moses to lead the charge (more on this in a minute), but his right-hand man was Aaron. He was the spokesperson to Pharaoh when Moses didn't feel qualified. He performed signs to the Israelites and was a mediator and intercessor. Aaron played a huge role in setting the Israelites free, but we tend to focus on Moses as the star of the story. That doesn't diminish Aaron's contribution, though.

Aaron achieved a servanthood calling. Sometimes, God asks us to help fulfill someone else's calling. I can't tell you how helpful it's been to have friends cheer me on and provide feedback while I write this book. Perhaps a friend needs financial support for a mission trip or simply another set of hands during a big event.

All callings are important. We may not get our name written in history as Aaron or Moses did, but that doesn't mean it's not impactful.

Seasonal callings

A calling for a period of time.

Sometimes God wants us to focus on something for a period of time. Then He pivots us to something else. It may be a clear path, or it may feel like a blindfolded pin-the-tail-on-the donkey step of faith. I'm currently in my third season, or "Phase Three" as I like to describe it. My first calling was to work diligently in the corporate world. Next up was as a stay-at-home mom. I was perfectly content in that role, but we learned at the beginning of this chapter that God had additional plans for me in mind. When we walk with God, we never know where He will take us and how long we will be there. We stay connected with Him and take the next step He asks us to take.

Macro callings

Larger-scale plans.

I list this one last because I wanted you to have a chance to consider the previous callings you've encountered. Recognize and honor where God has called you and whom you've blessed in the meantime, without qualifying your success by the size of your calling.

But back to our adventures of Moses. Moses, a Hebrew raised by Egyptians, killed an Egyptian and then ran for his life. He was leading a quiet life, tending to his flock, when God appeared to him in a flaming bush that did not burn to ashes. Through that burning bush, God announced to Moses that he was to rescue the Israelites from Egypt during this encounter. Talk about a macro calling.

Maybe God won't appear to you through a flaming bush, but have you ever gotten that fire in your heart that you are to do something big? Start a nonprofit. Go on a mission trip. Change careers. Start a family. Has your heart ever burned for an issue or a cause? What keeps you up at night? If you can't identify a macro calling right now, I bet God has you focusing on the other callings listed above. But keep your heart open and your eyes on the horizon for any large-scale callings He may be preparing for you.

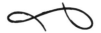

Admittedly, this truth of taking care of our bodies to fulfill our callings can get muddy. Joining my son at his favorite restaurant Whataburger (a Texas-based fast-food chain whose menu screams extra, super, and grease) does not change my short-term ability to fulfill my purpose. I can still write. I can still podcast. I can still train clients. I can even still record fitness videos, though I might be sporting all black to hide the guaranteed bloat. So, if I can still fulfill these callings, why not join him more often?

I don't think I need to tell you that repeated Whataburger visits over time would impair my ability to live out my calling. Even if my body composition didn't change, my heart, blood vessels, and organs would not thrive.

When I occasionally join my son at Whataburger, I'm not impeding any long-term objectives. Even if I have physical goals like increasing strength or losing weight, one single-combo-with-cheese-no-onion will not derail these targets. I'll say it again because that's a little mini rule that may not have its own chapter title but bears repeating: your long-term health goals will not be unmet if you eat fast food one time. But don't miss those last two words: one time. If you're trying to lose fifteen pounds in two months (a reasonable goal), receiving your meal through your car window once or twice will not push you back by another two months. Repeated drive-thru trips? Yes.

Part of my journey includes connecting the foods I'm eating to how my body interacts with them. Sometimes an entire meal will affect me; other times a single ingredient can. Most times I avoid these items, but not always (hence the added cheese in both the burger and omelet). It's a delicate balancing act that encourages me to think in both a short-term and long-term fashion, not unlike the various callings we have.

I'd like to tell you that since that lesson my pastor taught so many years ago, I've been able to keep my focus on what I'm called to do and off the size of my hips. The truth is I still wrestle this a lot more than I'd like to admit. I'm working on that (my attitude, not the size of my hips).

I'd also like to tell you I successfully achieve all my callings by taking care of my body. Just like those pancakes kept me from enjoying a few precious hours with my son, I've hindered my body in other ways. Overexercising in my thirties left me so spent I turned into a less-than-lovely mom and wife by the end of the day. A week ago I couldn't figure out why I needed afternoon naps; it turns out sugar was the culprit. And it pains me to admit there have been times I haven't been able to help a friend because my foggy head and tired body just didn't have the energy.

Your body does not work for you. It was given to us to glorify God, love and serve others, and fulfill the many types of callings God gives us. The apostle Paul teaches us this in 1 Corinthians 6:19–20:

> *Do you not know that your bodies are temples of the Holy Spirit, who is in you, whom you have received from God? You are not your own; you were bought at a price. Therefore honor God with your bodies.*

Our body, our temple, should honor God and His desire for us in all we do. (Or we should at least try. Lord knows I don't live up to it all the time.)

As for our callings, they change. Some are big, some are small. Some are long-term and some are short-term. But one thing they all have in common: our bodies need to be prepared for whatever God has for us.

The Simple Take:
Your body has a God-ordained purpose, but it's not always a huge, life-changing one. We can also have smaller, daily callings like creative callings, servanthood callings, and seasonal callings. What's important is that we are taking care of our body so we can execute these when we are asked.

Spend some time in prayer and thought about your callings. Write down examples of how you may feel called in each of the five areas.

Micro: mom+dad

Creative: entertaining

Servanthood: PTO to school,

Seasonal:

Macro energy at night to serve family w/ connection time

CHAPTER THREE

Do unto others. Period.

I deeply cherish my college girlfriends. Several years ago, we gathered for our annual girls' get-together. Most of us were done having babies, and as many women do, we were lamenting over the way bearing children affected our bodies. One of my friends confided in her plan to one day have a full mommy makeover. "I'm getting the whole shebang," she said. "A little suck, a little tuck, a little nip."

Obviously, cosmetic surgeries and procedures are a personal choice. I am not here to address that. What I found powerful and impactful was the response by the rest of the girls. She immediately experienced a laddering of compliments and body positivity. Some focused on her inner beauty, some focused on her outer beauty, and others reminded her how proportionate she is. There was no shaming of the decision she planned to make; it was just an opportunity to tell her how we saw her.

What would happen if I asked those same girls (myself included) who were heaping praise to look at themselves in the same light? Give me ten females in a lineup, and I can effortlessly pick out something beautiful about them. We easily see the beautiful creation God produced in others. But turn that around on myself, and it's a different story. I'm quick to see stretch marks, cellulite, and elevens between my eyebrows.

I'm working on reframing my thoughts to see myself as I see others. The journey isn't easy. Just like setting new health habits takes time and intentionality, so does self-positivity. Sometimes I'm great at this, and other times I find myself lifting and poking and sucking all the different ways I think my body needs to be lifted, minimized, and sucked.

Jesus commanded us to "*do to others as you would have them do to you*" in Luke 6:31. This is easy to remember most of the time. When I'm standing in line to check out my groceries, I enjoy letting someone in front of me who just has two items. I tip generously and look people in the eye.

But talking to myself like I talk to my friends? That's a lot harder. Why is this? Maybe one reason is we are taught at an early age to be humble. We are taught to love others. To be kind to others. We've grown up with such an emphasis on others that we forget to do the same for ourselves. We forget that self-care is part of caring for others.

The apostle Mark writes of the time a teacher of the law asked Jesus which commandment was most important. Jesus replied:

> *The most important one is this: hear, O Israel: "The Lord our God, The Lord is one. Love the Lord your God with all your heart and with all your soul and with all your mind and with all your strength." The second is this: "Love your neighbor as yourself." There is no commandment greater than these.*

Mark 12:29–31

This passage is probably not new to you. Love God. Love others. Simple enough. But don't forget the last two words: *as yourself*. We need to take care of our bodies, minds, and souls so we can best love others. Consider these approaches to learning to love and speak to ourselves better.

Evaluate the words you are telling yourself

If you're like me, you've seen the words "the power of positive thinking" for so long and so often you glaze over them. You may have even seen them plastered on an inspirational poster in your high school library. Right next to it was the kitten hanging onto the rope, proclaiming, "Hang in there!" It's easy to understand why we gloss over these words without much thought. But don't discount the power of positive thinking.

Now we have science that proves its power. Just like scientific evidence demonstrates the benefits of strength training and moving in different ways, brain science supports the benefits of positive thinking. *Psychology Today* reports that focused, repetitive mental activity can affect changes in your brain's structure, wiring, and capabilities.[1]

In other words, you can actually train your brain to be more positive. Still, I have a hard time quantifying positive thinking. I'm a numbers girl at heart. I like data, especially the kind that supports something I'm being told to do. If that's you too, consider this:

- Do you have a family history of heart disease? Try thinking more positively, and you'll be one-third less likely to have a heart attack or other cardiovascular event within five to twenty-five years than those with a more negative outlook.[2]
- A randomized control trial proved even fake smiling (and obviously real smiling) has its benefits: it reduces your heart rate and blood pressure during stressful situations.[3]
- A study out of Scotland revealed that positivity and physical health are positively correlated.[4] When test subjects rated higher on a positivity scale, they reported fewer physical symptoms on a scale listing stress, pain, anxiety, and depression.

The more I learn about the brain, the more I realize I have so much to learn. But this is one thing I do know: our thoughts matter. Thinking positive thoughts trains my brain to be more positive. Give yourself the same positive attributes you provide to your friends.

Kick out your obnoxious roommate

Not literally, if you do indeed have an obnoxious roommate. Well, maybe kick her out. But what I'm referring to are the negative thoughts invading our life that author and columnist Arianna Huffington terms "obnoxious roommates."[5] They do more than just annoy us.

Just like you can retrain your brain to be more positive, repeated negative thoughts are harmful as well:

- They can cause changes in neural connections that are associated with depression and anxiety.[6]
- One study showed that mice with high anxiety are prone to develop autoimmune diseases and have high levels of a protein called Immuno-moodulin.[7]
- Regularly worrying about the future and dwelling on the past saw larger drops in cognition and more harmful brain proteins than those who didn't do this, according to a study published by the *Alzheimer's & Dementia* journal.[8]

Kicking out a roommate is easier said than done. So is stopping those negative thoughts. The difference is you have full control over those negative thoughts. If you find yourself creating those negative neural pathways more often than you want, consider adopting a mantra of sorts that combats those negative thoughts with a positive response. Find a scripture that speaks to you or a quote that is general enough to apply in most situations but offers enough grace, gratitude, or grit to get yourself through. I asked my Facebook community to share some of theirs. If you need inspiration, I bet they won't mind if you borrow one:

- I am my own sunshine.
- Faith over fear.
- This too shall pass.
- I can do hard things.
- I choose joy.
- Jesus, you'll fix it.

And the crowd favorite is the apostle Paul's words at the end of Philippians 4:13: "*I can do all things through Him who gives me strength.*"

Harvard Medical School recommends these strategies for dealing with a negative thought life:[9]

- Recognize the problem.
- Identify new strategies.
- Set a limit on how long you allow yourself to focus on negative thoughts and worries.
- Put it in perspective.
- Adopt brain-healthy habits (which are pretty much the same as the physically healthy ones we discuss in this book).
- Seek help.

To reiterate that last point, getting help from a licensed counselor is a path to mental health progress. One of my podcast guests, Briana Leach, a Licensed Professional Counselor, educated me on the importance of not only reparative therapy but also preventative therapy. Just like I take my boys to well-child appointments and get a mammogram every year, stepping into a counselor's office before a crisis can help manage one better. Taking care of your mental health helps you to love others to your fullest extent. You can't pour into others if your cup is empty. It's hard to love others when you haven't given that same love and care to yourself.

Incorporate self-care into your calendar

The awareness of self-care is growing. This is a good thing. Unfortunately, it's sometimes hard to execute. I've had multiple conversations with podcast guests about self-care, each affirming the benefits. Yet if I'm honest, I still find it difficult.

If I can kill two birds with one stone and call something self-care *and* productive, it happens. Painting my toenails. Check. Taking a walk. Yep. Reading a book (if it's for an upcoming podcast guest). Affirmative.

But doing something simply for the sake of filling my soul? That's a harder sell. Reading a lighthearted fiction book while eating lunch feels scandalous. Absorbing the sun's warm rays on a spring day feels like wasting time.

Author and coach Elizabeth Barbour provides an abundance of self-care ideas in her book *Smart Self-Care for Busy Women.* She writes: *"Self-care is about exercising your voice, connecting with your power, and making choices in alignment with who you really are and how you want to live your life with intention."*[10] Depending on how God made you, self-care can take various forms. Here are a few ideas:

- Meditate (more on this below).
- Sit outside with no agenda.
- Walk (leisurely, not a power walk!).
- Take a bath.
- Declutter.
- Create art.
- Turn off screens.
- Read a book.
- Stretch.
- Find a way to move to keep your body strong and healthy.
- Fuel your body with God's foods
- Rest.
- Do something that brings you joy: reading, lunch with friends, or a date night with your spouse
- Give grace to the body in the mirror that doesn't look exactly how you want it to.

If you need self-care, here's a simple challenge: Choose one item from the list above, or create your own. Right now, put this book down, grab your calendar, and schedule it in today or tomorrow. Yes, I'm serious. If we don't schedule it in, chances are it won't happen. Or as author Dr. Saundra Dalton-Smith teaches in her book

Sacred Rest, *"Don't expect others to give you permission to take care of yourself."*[11]

Still unconvinced? Imagine your friend whose days are full and stressful. She never quite feels like she's getting everything done, and what does get done never feels like enough. Sometimes she has emotional breakdowns. One morning the two of you are texting. She confides she's taking an afternoon off to sit outside with a favorite beverage and novel she's been wanting to try but hasn't had the time.

You insert the clapping emojis into the text. Maybe even a little celebration hat. "Yes! Good for you! You deserve it!"

She does deserve it. So do you. Chances are, you are that friend whom others recognize needs a break. Take the initiative to treat yourself like your friend would and schedule that time to take care of yourself. If you encourage your friend to do that, you should too.

Consider starting your self-care with meditation

You may be tired of hearing of meditation. It seems like the latest buzzword that everyone is talking about. Or perhaps it just seems too hard or new agey for you. Yes, it's hard. Asking my brain to focus on one thing for more than a few seconds is like asking a toddler to sit quietly through church. While not impossible, it's an enormous challenge.

Meditation comes in many forms but is intended to promote focus and a heightened state of awareness. A common approach is simply sitting upright with your eyes closed and focusing on breathing. This is my tactic. I often use an app to guide me through it to prevent the aforementioned hyperactive thought pattern.

And before you dismiss it as too new age, remember we see examples of this throughout the Good Book. Isaac meditates in a field

(Gen. 24:63), the Lord tells Joshua to meditate on the Book of the Law (Josh. 1:8), and the psalmists mention meditation many times. I'm motivated by Psalm 104:35: *"May my meditation be pleasing to Him, as I rejoice in the Lord."*

I love it when science and scripture clearly align. We now have insight into God's intricate work through science and research and understand how beneficial this age-old practice is. Meditation:

- Reduces stress by lowering cortisol[12]
- Controls anxiety, depression, and pain[13]
- Reduces negative thoughts[14]
- Lengthens attention span
- May help fight addictions
- Improves sleep
- Decreases blood pressure
- Maintains a healthy gut microbiome[15]

Lately, I've been trying to meditate early in the afternoon. ("Trying" is the operative word.) When I do, my brain feels lighter and clearer. I find I have more energy to get through the day. My chest, which tends to store my stress, releases and melts to the ground, just like the app's gentle voice guides. One might think those are enough benefits to stay consistent. Yet I still talk myself out of taking the ten minutes in the name of being productive elsewhere.

If you're interested in trying meditation, there are several apps and even YouTube videos that offer guided meditation. I use one myself, but as I mentioned, sometimes I don't want to take a full ten minutes. Here's one way, a hack if you will, that enables me to practice mediation in microdoses. I set a timer for one minute...sixty seconds. As I breathe in, I say to myself "I am," and as I breathe out, I say "calm." It tends to help prevent the thoughts from ping-ponging around. Dr. Len Kravitz recommends this approach in his book *HIIT Your Limit: High-Intensity Interval Training for Fat Loss, Cardio,* and *Full Body Health*. Yes, even a book on high-intensity exercise promotes meditation. You can try other mantras as well. Find a few words from scripture or other life-giving words to focus on. Sometimes I say the words "breath of" as I inhale and "life" as I exhale. (A nod to Genesis 2:7 *"Then the Lord God formed a man from the dust of the ground and breathed into his nostrils the breath of life, and the man became a living being."*) Whatever words you choose, simply sit with your eyes closed and say them as you focus on your breath entering and leaving your body. Try it for one minute at first, and extend your time as you become more comfortable.

Taking the time to focus on my breath is an essential part of taking care of myself. The investment is worth it.

Evaluate how you're spending your time

How much time do you spend with your Creator? Not the quick prayers that resemble texts to God, but true, meaningful conversations with Him. Invest time with Jesus. I am a better wife, mother, and human being when I get up early to drink coffee and spend time with Jesus. Period. And my day just seems off when I don't. How I spend my time changes, but my why does not. Sometimes I immerse myself in a Beth Moore study, other times I read the Word and journal, and sometimes I read a YouVersion Bible plan and watch the daily video stories.

Author Jennie Allen writes that *"real, connected, intimate time with Jesus is the very thing that grows our faith, shifts our mind, brings about revival in our souls, and spreads to others."*[16]

Also, invest in time with your people. The emotional benefits they provide are immeasurable. As Dr. Bessel van der Kolk writes in his groundbreaking book *The Body Keeps the Score*, *"Being able to feel safe with other people is probably the single most important aspect of mental health; safe connections are fundamental to meaningful and satisfying lives."*[17]

I experienced a version of this during the summer of 2020 when COVID-19 put us all in an upheaval. While my husband is truly my best friend, there's something about girlfriends that offer a different sacred element. I had dropped my son off at camp an hour-and-a-half away and drove a little farther to meet one of my closest college friends at an outdoor park. She stepped out of her car, and we looped masks around our ears and embraced. I wept. All the anxiety and stress I'd been experiencing had a safe landing place on her shoulder. The next hour-and-a-half refreshed my soul and mental health. But it took an investment of time on both of our parts to make it happen.

On a closer level, I did this with my local friends as well. While my emotional health suffered during the pandemic, I truly believe it would have been worse without investing the time to walk with friends. I even made a new friend during this period of isolation, whom you'll meet in the next chapter.

Taking time away from your family and responsibilities to see safe, cherished friends is not selfish. It's an element of taking care of yourself and essential to your mental health.

Remember "it" happens

I tend to be a positive person. In general, it serves me well, though I'm learning looking at the bright side of things is not always helpful when dealing with the hard stuff. My life has many examples of times I tried to make someone feel better when all they really needed was someone to sit with them.

If you're in one of those spaces where you just need someone to sit with you, I hear you. I see you. Life happens. Stuff happens. (If we were enjoying a coffee together face-to-face, I'd use a different word.) In 2020 alone, we witnessed the loss of life and jobs, racial injustice, and higher stress than many of us have ever experienced. Some of our friendships changed due to polarizing politics. But maybe part of your story goes much farther back than 2020. Perhaps God hasn't given you that spouse or child you always thought you would have. A medical condition altered your life. Someone close to you died unexpectedly due to suicide, and it changed your entire trajectory.

Traumatic events, big and small, affect our bodies. We lose self-awareness, are startled and frustrated easily, have disturbed sleep, and lose pleasure from food.[18]

Cortisol, a hormone secreted when stressed, continues to release long after the danger has passed. Thousands of years ago, danger may have been a wild animal chasing you. Now it's more insidious. It's grief, addiction, money concerns, and infidelity. But our bodies still respond the same. That excess cortisol impacts our mental health, heart, memory, and digestion.

What does this have to do with loving and taking care of ourselves? Part of this process is honoring the space we are in. This book is not intended to be a quick fix or a guarantee of anything. (Except grace. Grace is always a guarantee.) As we enter Part 2 shortly, I hope you feel empowered to do what works for you and leave the rest. The various tools and resources mentioned throughout this book will be here waiting for you when you want to try something else. But be sure to take the grace with you.

If all else fails...

Here's a radical thought: Perhaps all this brain science is catching up to what Paul wrote to the Philippians two thousand years ago.

> *Finally, brothers and sisters, whatever is true, whatever is noble, whatever is right, whatever is pure, whatever is lovely, whatever is admirable—if anything is excellent or praiseworthy—think about such things.*

Philippians 4:8

True. Noble. Right. Pure. Lovely. Admirable. Excellent. Praiseworthy. Think about such things.

I am wonderfully made in God's image. So are you. When I intentionally think excellent thoughts about myself, I'm honoring God and His work in me.

Some of that self-care comes with being kind to ourselves.

Take care of yourself today. Give yourself grace today. Love yourself today. And do your body and brain a favor and say a few nice things about yourself.

The Simple Take:
Use your best friend as a litmus test when you're talking to and taking care of yourself. Treat yourself with the same kindness you'd give to her. If you wouldn't say it to her, don't say it to yourself.

Let's start taking care of ourselves by paying attention to our thoughts and brain health. Fill out this form today, or download one to print off for daily use in the resource guide.

Three things my body did well yesterday:

1. walk
Pure barre - strength
Sleeping

2.

3.

One way I will honor my body today:

1. walking
reading

☐ Meditate

CHAPTER FOUR

She has
THE
perfect body

Author's note: *I enter this conversation and sacred space humbly with the highest amount of respect I can offer. The terminology I use, particularly Black, is meant with deep reverence and a result of many leaders declaring, "Just call me Black." I also recognize the Black community is not a monolith, and I am not foolish enough to think this chapter applies to all Black women's bodies.*

My first job provided me an unusual perk of having a first-floor window office. That sounds much fancier than my job really was; it was simply a result of space configuration. Every day around 11:00 a.m., I'd watch the foot traffic pick up as people headed to the diner next door.

One day, I found myself gazing out the window when I should have been working. I noticed a group of coworkers presumably headed to lunch. One woman stood out to me. She appeared to have the kind of confidence I could only hope for. She donned a figure-shaping ribbed dress that displayed her curvaceous figure. The bright orange dress complimented her dark skin in the most perfect way possible. She was stunning.

I knew I would never be brave enough to wear a dress that snug. And while I admired her confidence, a part of me was happy to let her enjoy her curves while I still tried to lose five pounds.

When I see a Black woman self-assured in her curves, I'm jealous. And curious. How is it that she can stand so confidently when part of the unwritten female code is to be unhappy with how we look? (Another rule to break!) Or is that just a white-woman thing? How can I get a piece of that confidence? How can I influence others to do the same?

My friend Camisha and I spend Saturday mornings walking. We initially met at one of my fitness classes. We paired up again a few months later when she accepted a call for a Black woman to participate in a six-week virtual race through Black Girls Run. This race was developed to promote racial reconciliation after the murder of George Floyd at the hands of police in 2020.

Our first time out, we had barely turned the corner from her house when Camisha and I began discussing politics. Over the next three miles, we also covered capitalism, health, and body image. You know, we kept it light. Though we didn't agree on everything, we were both open to exploring other thoughts beyond our own. And in a way only God can orchestrate, Camisha was a fellow writer working on her first book.

Through our friendship, Camisha has granted me the safety and grace to ask uncomfortable questions regarding Black body image. I can't express my gratitude enough for this.

I've also been on my own exploration by listening and learning from the Black community for several years. As I've reflected on my journey, learned more about the racial history of body image, and had many conversations with Camisha about it, I've discovered a few spaces to sit and grow in. I'd like to share these spaces and growth opportunities with you.

If you are white and this is your first time hearing some of the discussion below, it may be uncomfortable. But I encourage you to lean in anyway. Just like my goal later in the next section is to break fitness and nutrition rules you may have heard, my goal in this section is to work together to shift our thinking about body ideals and where they come from.

Recognize and remember that all bodies, colors, and shapes are created in the image of God

We can't get out of the first chapter of the first book of the Bible without learning that we are all created in the image of God (Gen. 1:27). When I think about the image of God, I think it's natural to envision what and who we know. My first visual is an old white man with a gray beard sitting atop the clouds. I suppose I can chalk that up to the children's Bibles and Vacation Bible School depictions that had the daunting task of explaining God to a three-year-old. Then my mind shifts to revered spiritual leaders many of us grew up with like Billy Graham and Pope John Paul II.

I now see more diversity in mainstream spiritual leaders. Thank you, Jesus, for that. Thank you for Beth Moore, Priscilla Shirer, the Most Reverend Michael Curry, and countless others who represent a broader image of God while teaching us about Him.

But when my mind filters down specifically to me and how I am created in God's image, I become narrow-minded. For some reason, I feel like in order to represent His image best, I need to be skinny. God is not only a skinny white woman. He's also curvy, short, tall, and all the colors of His people. I can't pretend to completely understand the complexities of all bodies, shapes, and skin colors being made in God's image. However, I do know when I stack my earthly understanding of bodies against the greatness of God, I will always underestimate Him.

God in the flesh, Jesus, likely had brown skin. Our Anglo culture has washed the melanin out of Him. He ministered to all bodies and races in His actions and parables. Are we seeing everybody, regardless of their melanin, as one made in the image of God? Maybe it's time we start recognizing the image of God in everyone and stop holding ourselves to the skinny-white-woman standard.

Our genetics and set point factor into our different sizes...and it's okay if they are different

If the image of God is in all of us, yet I'm uncomfortable wanting more curves than I have, then where does that leave me?

It leaves me becoming comfortable that both my body and that of the woman walking by my office window are acceptable. In fact, it can give me confidence that the shape my body gravitates to is the right shape for me when I move and eat the foods God gave me. And a curvy body that fuels well and moves is also the right shape for others, including the Black woman in the orange dress.

Consider the set point theory. The "set point" theory states that our bodies have a preset weight baseline hardwired into our DNA. According to this theory, our weight and how much it changes from that set point might be limited. The theory says that some of us have higher weight set points than others, and our bodies fight to stay within these ranges.[1]

I know I'm around my set point because I'm virtually the same size I was when I got married at age twenty-two. If I completely exhale every bit of air in my lungs and suck in my gut, my sister can still zip up my wedding dress. Well, almost. She needs to fold over a bit of skin along my spine as well. Maybe this isn't a great example. Yes, I've gained ten-ish pounds, but who's counting? I've also carried two babies, more than doubled my age, and increased my muscle tone. The point is I'm still basically the same size as the chubby-cheeked twenty-two-year-old baby who said "I do." It just ain't changing much.

If my body became significantly more curvy than it is, it probably wouldn't function as well. I've seen this in my blood pressure, which tends to creep up around the holidays when I'm not exactly fueling my best. I also get woken up by my husband telling me to roll over because I'm snoring.

God created my body uniquely. When I fill it with the foods He provides, move it in a way that brings me joy, and speak words of life to
myself, I create deposits of confidence. That confidence reminds me
that I'm taking care of my body so I can do what God is calling me to
do, not so it will look a certain way.

It feels like a juxtaposition to say I admire curves but in the same
breath declare I don't want to be more curvy. However, maybe these
can exist in the same space because God created us differently. I
shouldn't compare my body to hers or vice versa. Doing so wouldn't
honor how we were both made.

Black women's body image does not begin and end with size

For three years, I was an ambassador to an athletic-wear company
that valued diversity, inclusivity, and high-quality clothes in which
to exercise. I met some incredible women through this organization
and am so grateful for my time as part of the team. One year I attended an ambassador retreat, where one Black speaker shared her
story of being a self-proclaimed big girl who had positively trans-
formed her health over the years. She dropped sixty pounds after a
health scare, settling into about 240 pounds and maintaining that
for several years. In the meantime, she completed marathons, tri-
athlons, and a slew of other physical accomplishments. She seemed
to have found her set point and was thriving in her body. She asked
if anyone had any questions. My white hand cautiously raised. "Was
there any discussion around body image growing up?"

I wasn't sure what her blank look meant at first. Eventually, she
responded, "Well, it just wasn't ever discussed. It wasn't an issue
because we never talked about size or weight."

I didn't know a nondiscussion of size or weight even existed. Many
of my white friends have a similar story to mine: I can't remember
a time growing up that I was happy with my body. It's a theme so

intricately threaded throughout our lives, most of us can't share a story of growing up where we don't bring up our body-image issues. And for Black women who have attended school or work in white spaces, I'm told by Black friends this may be their story as well. (Jesus, help us all.)

Camisha tells me that blank look spoke volumes. It could have masked any of these thoughts:

- While thinness has always been a goal of mine, this doesn't necessarily hold true for Black women. For some, a bigger body might demonstrate health and strength. An article in the *Journal of African American Studies* reports that Black women accept a wider range of body shapes, even if their BMIs classify them as overweight and obese.[2] You will soon learn my thoughts on the BMI chart. Spoiler alert, I give it two thumbs down.

- Black women have a whole host of other physical issues they deal with. How dark or light is their skin? How curly is their natural hair?

- Black women may deal with more-pressing issues than what their body looks like. From being less likely to be promoted in their careers and to have access to benefits like paid leave—in conjunction with childcare costs taking over half their income—to being more likely to be denied home loans,[3] they may not have the headspace to fret about body image.

- Or, it may be a both/and situation. That blank look may have been a calculation of how deep to answer my question.

It's hard to know what the blank look meant, but we can't ignore the complexities surrounding it.

The thin ideal is rooted in white supremacy and racism

Last week I pulled out the scale. The digital numbers displayed 146.4 (as if that .4 pound matters). On my five-foot-four frame, this is at the high end of what's considered normal. I've already shared that

I'm pretty much at my set point. Yet it's taken me years to absolve myself of the wasted energy to wish I was thinner. I attribute my healing to a mindset shift in why I take care of my body, which we will discuss in the next chapter, but I'd like to present one more idea I've recently learned: *American beauty culture originated in white supremacy.*

Shocked? So was I.

Some activists and researchers blame a chart called the Quetelet Index. It was developed in the mid-nineteenth century to study human traits as they related to crime and mortality. Mr. Quetelet, the developer, was not a doctor or health expert of any kind, but was intent on figuring out what the "ideal man" looked like. He searched for a model of perfection, evaluating proportions, conditions, and disease. Anything differing from that would be considered a "monstrosity." His data came primarily from white European men and was not intended to be used to measure a person's health or wellness. Later, in the twentieth century, health and life insurance companies adopted this Quetelet Index. It was renamed in 1972. Can you guess what this height-to-weight ratio is called now? If you guessed the Body Mass Index (BMI), you are correct.[4]

So how is the BMI rooted in white supremacy? Well, for one, the chart was originally based off of white European men. It imagined "ideal" Caucasians and didn't consider other factors like gender or ethnicity. This is important as we understand our overall health. While BMI variations are now made for gender, ethnicity remains unaccounted for. Yet, as our research and access to data has grown, we understand more. For example, a large 2003 study in the *Journal of the American Medical Association* reported that higher BMIs tend to be more optimal for Black people. But the BMI chart doesn't take that into consideration. It's simply a chart of numbers and ratios.

Another reason for fat fear is the equation of thinness to elitism. This began as a social distinction that favored thinness over fatness for those at the top of the social hierarchy. Author Sabrina Strings writes in *Fearing the Black Body* that:

> *scholars have identified the United States as the country in which the pro-thin, anti-fat bias was gaining strength among elite, morally upright white Americans (especially women) by the nineteenth century and crystallized into a mainstream position by the early twentieth century.*[5]

This last point sickens me to write but is worth mentioning to expand our understanding. Art, philosophy, and science have historically used the image of the fat Black woman to depict savagery and barbarianism. This diminished Black women and drove the symbol of the ideal body as, you guessed it, a skinny white woman.[6]

To be clear, I'm not knocking skinny people. Thin women exist in every culture. Some of these thin women are healthy on the inside while some, unfortunately, are not. Healthy curvy women exist in every culture too. My hope for this chapter is to open our eyes to where this thin ideal came from so that we can begin thinking about what the image of God means to us.

While I was soliciting help for women's experiences growing up in different cultures, one generous Black woman responded in a way I didn't expect but absolutely loved. Her words capture the essence of my discussions surrounding how we view our bodies:

> *To me, the "ideal" body image for Black women is self-confidence. We tend to look in the mirror with resigned acceptance of who we are and how we look relative to the world around us. We should [instead] look in the mirror with eyes of self-love, and they will reflect one's own "ideal" body image.*

I have a lot of research and learning left to do. I also know this discussion only scratches the surface. This chapter's resource contains much of the research I used for this section as well as other books and podcasts that have impacted me. Our Black American brothers and sisters have experienced oppression and racism for over four hundred years. Their bodies have been underrepresented, underappreciated, commodified, and objectified. I'm not naive enough to think we can change things quickly. But perhaps we start with the same foundation of what I need to work on: recognizing, treating, and loving every body as made perfect in the image of God. There is not one perfect body.

The Simple Take:
The perfect body simply doesn't exist. It's time we
start recognizing the image of God in all bodies by
recognizing and loving the differences He made.

If you're interested in learning more about racial justice and reconciliation, or have questions about Black culture, consider the following resources I've found helpful.

Books (in alphabetical order by author)

Uncomfortable Conversations with a Black Man
by Emmanuel Acho

White Awake: An Honest Look at What It Means to Be White by Daniel Hill

Be the Bridge: Pursuing God's Heart for Racial Reconciliation
by Latasha Morrison

Loves...Regardless: A Love and Spirit Offering to Black Women
by Rev. Donna Owusu-Ansah

Fearing the Black Body: The Racial Origins of Fat Phobia
by Sabrina Strings

Under Our Skin: Getting Real About Race—and Getting Free from the Fears and Frustrations That Divide Us
by Benjamin Watson with Ken Peterson

Podcasts

Smartest Person in the Room with Laura Tremaine: "Bias" Series

For the Love with Jen Hatmaker: "For the Love of Black Lives" Series

Food Heaven Podcast with Wendy Lopez and Jessica Jones:
A multimedia platform founded by two Black registered dietitians and BFFs. They help people transform the way they eat and find joy in food through the practice of intuitive eating and body respect.

CHAPTER FIVE

I can tell you're healthy by looking at you

Several years ago, I huddled on the bleachers of my son's basketball game. I can't tell you exactly when this was because he's been playing basketball practically since he was old enough to say the word "basketball." I was chatting with a group of women, and the conversation turned to whatever fitness class I was teaching at the time. "You should come and try it!" I said, looking one girl in the eye. "I bet you'd love it."

I felt an energy shift. I could tell I'd misstepped. Yes, I invited the woman sitting next to me. But I completely ignored and failed to offer the same to another mom nearby. The mom whose larger size made me think she wasn't into fitness.

I don't know if I've uttered this chapter's title, but I can tell you I'm guilty of assuming the opposite. To my deep regret, my mind has assumed someone is not healthy based on her size. I know better now. God and my journey have shifted me away from assuming anything about someone's health based on their size. However, I admit I'm still ashamed of moments in the past when I have.

Unfortunately, it's easy to get caught up in visually assessing someone's health based on their size. We already discussed my disdain for the BMI chart. Will you indulge me a bit more while I complain about it? Merriam-Webster.com defines weight as the "*force with which a body is attracted toward the earth.*"[1] Total weight does not distinguish between muscle mass, fat mass, or hydration levels. The BMI does not take this into account either. Google "professional athletes who have a high BMI." You'll be shocked to see who qualifies as "clinically obese." Their high muscle mass contributes to a higher weight, yet this is not accounted for in the BMI. And if you still need convincing, remember this: There's no BMI in the Bible. God never set boundaries on how we are supposed to look, only that we treat our body as a temple of the Holy Spirit.

If we can't determine health visually or through a BMI chart, how can we figure out our personal health index? Unfortunately, there's no formula. Let's change that to "fortunately, there's no formula." It isn't a single-dimension metric that we can pass or fail, like a high school chemistry test. In fact, our individual body chemistry dictates much of our overall health. Consider some of the following.

Blood metrics

When you visit your internal medicine physician for your annual checkup, she probably has you donate several vials of blood. Your blood is analyzed and sent back to her for review. She will look at various metrics like blood sugar, cholesterol profile, vitamin D, and thyroid, liver, iron, and kidney function. As she is your doctor, and I am not, I will let the two of you determine what your blood is telling you about your body's health. But rest assured, those little red vials can reveal so much.

Blood pressure metrics

It's not called the "silent killer" for nothing. If your blood pressure is elevated and your doctor wants to talk about how to manage it, listen to her. High blood pressure can create a stroke, vision loss, heart failure, heart attack, kidney disease/failure, and sexual disfunction. Do what you need to do to get this number at a level that your doctor is comfortable with.

If you've developed high blood pressure and the thought of medicating yourself bothers you, perhaps this gives you comfort: every morning, I pop not one but two pills to keep my blood pressure under control. Am I thrilled about this? Not in the least bit. Am I doing my part to manage it? Absolutely. Turns out that even with daily exercise and a whole-foods, plant-heavy diet, I still can't control it. I shove my ego aside and swallow those two pills.

I'm irritated that I have to resort to medicine, but this is why I do: *it's not about me.* I make too many positive decisions for my body not to help it where it needs it. My boys and husband deserve their mom and wife around for as long as possible. Your people deserve this as well. If you and your doctor feel like you've made all the lifestyle adjustments you can and that number isn't dropping, just take the pills.

Body metrics

I don't want to focus too heavily on this element because the body metrics are truly just one aspect of our health. But for the sake of being comprehensive, here we go.

Measure your waist-to-hip ratio or waist circumference. Either one is acceptable.

The World Health Organization recommends a waist-to-hip ratio of .85 or less.[2] Not sure what yours is? Grab a fabric measuring tape. Measure around your belly button (waist) and around the largest part of your buttocks and hips. Divide the waist measurement by the hip.

You may also measure your waist circumference. The American Heart Association and the National Heart, Lung, and Blood Institute recommend your waist to be less than thirty-five inches around.[3] This measurement is at the smallest point in your waist (as opposed to around your belly button in the waist-to-hip ratio). I'm not sure why we can't be consistent in the measuring points, but I am merely the messenger.

In people who are not overweight, having a large waist may mean that they are at higher risk of health problems than someone with a trim waist. The Nurses' Health Study, one of the largest and longest studies to date that has measured abdominal obesity, looked at the relationship between waist size and death from heart disease, cancer, or any cause in middle-aged women. At the start of the study, all 44,000 study volunteers were healthy, and all of them measured their waist size and hip size. After sixteen years, women who had reported the highest waist sizes (thirty-five inches or higher) had nearly *double the risk* of dying from heart disease, compared to women who had reported the lowest waist sizes (less than twenty-eight inches).[4]

Women in the group with the largest waists had a similarly high risk of death from cancer or any cause, compared with women with the smallest waists. The risks increased steadily with every added inch around the waist.

What is it about abdominal fat that makes it a strong marker of disease risk? The fat surrounding the liver and other abdominal organs, so-called visceral fat, is metabolically active. It releases fatty acids, inflammatory agents, and hormones that ultimately lead to higher LDL cholesterol, triglycerides, blood glucose, and blood pressure.[5]

I'd also like to take this opportunity to remind you that our genetics will play a part in where we store fat. You may be strong, agile, healthy, and well functioning but still uncomfortable with that waist circumference. Some things just aren't fair. A friend pointed out how lucky pear-shaped women are in this regard. I agree. But this is also why we have a host of metrics to evaluate our health and *we can't tell if someone is healthy by looking at them.*

Alternatively, if you're lucky enough to have low body metrics of waist-to-hip ratio or waist circumference but receive most of your food through the window of your car, please don't fool yourself. Just like we can't assume one's health based on her larger size, it's unfair to assume someone's healthy if she's thin or underweight. Her size doesn't necessarily reflect healthy habits.

It may also be that her body is fighting something fierce on the inside and it's manifesting as weight loss. Cancer, Crohn's disease, hyperthyroidism, and diabetes can all cause the scale to drop. I've never heard anyone declare they embraced cancer because it helped them lose weight. Similarly, a sudden increase in weight (without an increase in cookies) may reflect other health issues like thyroid issues or polycystic ovary syndrome, so if you've noticed a big swing one way or the other, please visit your doctor.

The body metrics are just one aspect in considering our health. Pay attention to them, but don't put full stock in them. And certainly don't let your scale dictate your health.

Sleep metrics

How well do you sleep? In my early twenties, I found myself in a stage of having the darnedest time falling asleep. I knew my body was tired because A) I'd worked a full day, and B) I hadn't slept well in weeks. Night after night, I'd lay in my bed witnessing my anxiety level increase as the potential hours for sleep decreased. After paying attention to what I was consuming, I realized the caffeine-infused peach-flavored tea I enjoyed with dinner was the culprit.

Classic forehead slap. I quit drinking my delicious tea and haven't had it since. And the sleep? It returned to normal. Aside from short periods of time when I can't nod off due to my brain working overtime, distress about a situation, or my belly getting me back for indulging in something it doesn't like (*darn you* baked Brie!), I am thankful to have quality sleep most nights.

I recognize this isn't the case for everyone. Some of our brains tend to solve the world's problems right when it's time to go to bed. Others nod off just fine but wake up at 3:00 a.m. for several hours.

The National Institutes of Health reports that numerous factors contribute to sleep disruption, ranging from lifestyle and environmental factors to sleep disorders and other medical conditions.[6] Normal healthy sleep is characterized by sufficient duration, good quality, appropriate timing and regularity, and the absence of sleep disturbances and disorders[7] like sleep apnea and restless legs syndrome. If this doesn't describe your overall sleep health, you may be having sleep issues.

This is the scary thing: when we lack sleep health, our short-term and long-term health suffers. In his book *Keep Sharp*, Dr. Sanjay Gupta teaches that *"a single night of inadequate sleep is enough to activate inflammatory processes in the body, especially in women for reasons we don't know yet."*[8]

Additionally, sleep disruption is associated with increased activity of the sympathetic nervous system.[9] Your sympathetic nervous system manages your "fight or flight" response. In essence, when your sleep is disturbed, your brain may be at risk of fighting off a threat or fleeing from an enemy, releasing adrenaline and cortisol.[10] This can also create metabolic effects, changes in circadian rhythms, and pro-inflammatory responses.

The Cleveland Clinic offers ten ways sleep deprivation affects your health:

1. Fatigue, low energy, and excessive sleepiness (no shock there)
2. Irritability
3. Neurological disturbances including blurred vision, memory lapses, poor reaction time, and drooping eyelids
4. Lowered immune system
5. In women: a higher likelihood to suffer coronary events (when sleeping less than seven hours per night)
6. Impaired glucose tolerance, or higher-than-normal blood sugar levels
7. Elevated cortisol ("the stress hormone")

8. Altered levels of key hormones like ghrelin, leptin, and cortisol (ghrelin activates hunger, and leptin communicates satiety)

9. Abnormal thyroid function and growth-hormone secretion

10. In children and teens: behavior problems, impaired learning, poor concentration, and decreased school performance[11]

If you're struggling with sleep, consider these tips from the Sleep Foundation:

1. Create a sleep-inducing bedroom. Choose quality bedding, limit lights, cultivate peace and quiet, and find a Goldilocks temperature: not too warm, not too cold.

2. Optimize your sleep schedule. Try to go to sleep and wake around the same time, keep naps to twenty minutes in the early afternoon, and get between seven and nine hours a night.

3. Create a prebedtime routine. Turn off screens, wind down for thirty minutes, and lower your lights.

4. Foster pro-sleep habits during the day. Get out in the sunlight, move, watch your caffeine and alcohol intake, and don't eat too late.[12]

Dr. Gupta also writes that "*sleep is the single most effective thing we can do to reset our brains and bodies, as well as increase a healthy life span.*"[13]

I'm going to say something a little controversial, but this is what I believe: *You can skip a workout to sleep.* Yes, you can. Listen to that incredible body and brain of yours. If you need to take an occasional day off to get some more zzz's, then do it. We will talk more about rest days in "No Rest for the Weary."

You probably don't need me to tell you how important sleep is. If you're experiencing ongoing sleep issues, please reach out to your doctor or a sleep specialist. You may be doing "all the right things," but if you're still watching the clock tick, it may be indicative of a deeper issue. Let the experts help you find your way back to quality zzzz's. Your health depends on it.

Mental metrics

In February 2020, I attended a podcast conference. If I'm honest, I attended with two goals, in this order: 1) learn new things about podcasting, and 2) meet other podcasters and become a guest on their shows.

As it often happens, God's plans did not line up nice and neat with mine. I received only one invitation to guest on another show. Instead, He placed key women and fellow podcasters in my path who not only have their own show but also are therapists. I walked away realizing I wanted, needed, to have a series on mental health on the podcast. These mental health professionals taught me the importance of recognizing my emotions' impact on my body and how they are intricately integrated. I'm not alone. As of this writing, some of the most downloaded episodes of the *Graced Health* podcast revolve around mental health, and I continue to invite professionals on the show to help me and my listeners learn more.

In other words, I can't run off the crazy. Sure, it can help mitigate it (and yes, studies prove this), but shoving all my issues into my running shoes or yoga pants may not be enough.

It doesn't matter what my body looks like on the outside. If my mind is a hot mess that snaps with a misloaded glass in the dishwasher, I'm not in an optimal place.

Let's say you have a friend who executes her food and exercise plan perfectly. She's nailing it. But she's cranky. All the time. And she won't go out to eat because it will derail her. She's anxious about her food and exercise and quite honestly not very much fun to be around. Would you describe this friend as healthy? Maybe she is physically, but from a mental health perspective, I'd argue no. All that stress and anxiety may do just as much damage as a fast-food No. 1 burger combo with cheese.

And if you need another reason to keep moving for your brain health, know this: movement helps prevent cognitive decline and helps maintain better processing skills in aging brains.[14]

Take care of your mental health. Revisit the ways we discussed this in "Do Unto Others. Period." And seek a therapist if you need to. Taking care of your brain helps all aspects of your body. They are all intertwined.

Functionality metrics

A study out of Europe[15] researched the predictors of longevity. Researchers asked, What determines how long we will live? If asked this question prior to reading the study, I might have suggested the answer lies somewhere between blood pressure, blood metrics, or even waist-to-hip ratio. I'd be wrong. Shockingly, the answer has to do with how well we can come to a standing position from being seated crisscross on the floor without using our hands or knees.*

What? You mean of all the medical tests out there, I just need to be able to get up off the ground easily? Apparently, yes. Think about all that goes into elevating your whole frame. You need core strength, flexible hip flexors, and strong quads and glutes to rise to a standing position. Your heart needs to be able to handle the exertion, and your blood pressure needs to adapt.

Generally speaking, it becomes harder for us to elevate off the floor as we age. Regardless if this is something you can achieve or not, you still want to be able to move throughout your day fluidly. Some of my functional metrics include:

- Not be winded after taking the stairs to tell my boys goodnight.

- Be able to crawl under the couch to retrieve my dog's bone. (How did it get there anyway?)
- Transfer the thirty pack of Costco bottled water to my cart, car, and home.
- Lug the forty-pound bags of salt from the pool supply store to my trunk, at which point I ask my boys to carry it in. (I get a little lazy.)
- Hike with anyone whenever and wherever I find elevation; Houston is as flat as a pancake.

All these are measures of my functional health. Regardless of the size of my body, if I can't function in any of the items above, I'm not running at full capacity. I'm not using my body as best as I can, and I'm certainly not at optimal energy.

Your body has a holistic way of telling you if you're healthy. One metric does not tell the whole story. We can't assess health by looking at a single metric, and we certainly can't tell just by looking at someone. Whatever size range your body falls in, it has several ways of communicating its overall health with you.

If you're like me and want to perform this test on your own, here are the specifics per "The Washington Post." Lower yourself to the floor, crisscross style, without bracing yourself with your hands, knees, arms, or sides of your legs. If you can stand back up without the aid of any of those body parts, you've scored a perfect ten (five for sitting, five for standing). You lose a point every time you support yourself with any of the listed appendages.

The Simple Take:
Visually assessing one's health never tells the whole story. A holistic assessment of metrics shown through blood work, blood pressure, waist circumference, sleep, mental health, and functionality will tell the full story.

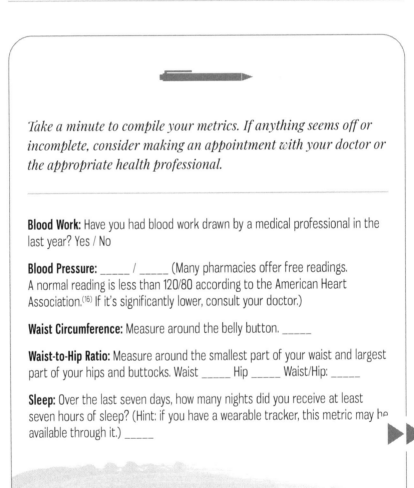

Take a minute to compile your metrics. If anything seems off or incomplete, consider making an appointment with your doctor or the appropriate health professional.

Blood Work: Have you had blood work drawn by a medical professional in the last year? Yes / No

Blood Pressure: _____ / _____ (Many pharmacies offer free readings. A normal reading is less than 120/80 according to the American Heart Association.[16] If it's significantly lower, consult your doctor.)

Waist Circumference: Measure around the belly button. _____

Waist-to-Hip Ratio: Measure around the smallest part of your waist and largest part of your hips and buttocks. Waist _____ Hip _____ Waist/Hip: _____

Sleep: Over the last seven days, how many nights did you receive at least seven hours of sleep? (Hint: if you have a wearable tracker, this metric may be available through it.) _____

Mental Health: Do you have any signs and symptoms of mental illness? If you've experienced any of the conditions below for longer than a month, it may be time to seek assistance from a mental health professional.

- Feeling sad or down
- Confused thinking or reduced ability to concentrate
- Excessive fears or worries, or extreme feelings of guilt
- Extreme mood changes of highs and lows
- Withdrawal from friends and activities
- Significant tiredness, low energy, or problems sleeping
- Detachment from reality (delusions), paranoia, or hallucinations
- Inability to cope with daily problems or stress
- Trouble understanding and relating to situations and to people
- Problems with alcohol or drug use
- Major changes in eating habits
- Sex-drive changes
- Excessive anger, hostility, or violence
- Suicidal thinking

Functional Health: On a scale of 1-10, how am I able to live out my day-to-day responsibilities without hurting myself or becoming overly tired?

1   2   3   4   5   6   7   8   9   10

PART TWO: GET 'ER DONE

Now that we've warmed up our mindset, it's time to break some health and fitness rules. These are the memes, T-shirts, and Pinterest images that make me cringe. It's time to quit letting a marketing campaign or Instagram feed dictate how successful we feel in our movement and eating habits.

Speaking of movement, I tend to use that word in place of "exercise" or "workout." Sometimes those latter words conjure up memories of unrelenting coaches or trainers. Maybe "exercise" is a reminder of an unused gym membership or feeling inadequate in that kickboxing class. Or perhaps it's a reminder of how many times you "have to work out" in a week. While I describe moving our body as all three words, I particularly appreciate the word "movement." Doesn't it just sound more joyful and freeing?

I hope you enjoy the resources throughout this section. If you're a visual learner or prefer to have printouts, remember to scan the QR code below to receive free access to the videos, recipes, and more.

CHAPTER SIX

I have to work off dessert

The statement "I have to work off dessert" has woven itself through my brain for so long it's practically white noise. Every bite of my four-year-old's Thomas the Train cupcakes, boxed-lunch oatmeal raisin cookie, and Twizzlers purchased between last period and my high school job received the same caveat: I have to work this off. I uttered those words so often they came to lack significant value. They became rote. Sometimes I actually did work the cookies off in that evening's kickboxing class. Other times I added another penny's worth of shame to my collection.

Sometimes I uttered these words to myself at the same time I indulged in the sugar before me:

- "My baby only turns three once; why not have a cupcake?"
- "Girls' Night Out is only once a month; pass a fork for the shared seven-layer cake."
- "The circus only comes once a year; of course I'll split a cotton candy with my kiddo."

The juxtaposition of indulgence and shame became so common that it eventually felt *normal*. How could I enjoy something without simultaneously feeling like I'd failed? Clearly, I had to work off that failure. I calculated the calories of that cake or cookie and made a mental note to make sure tomorrow's workout included the equal amount of time needed to offset that intake. Even better if I could get an extra workout in.

One of the first tenets I learned in weight management (which was always the impetus of my crazy) was "calories in, calories out." My body requires a certain amount of energy, otherwise known as calories. Intake too many calories, and they are stored as fat. Burn more calories than I consume, and my body will pull from the fat stores to find energy.

Sounds simple enough, right? Sort of. It's a significantly simplified version of my body's food utilization. "Calories in vs. calories out" doesn't take into consideration the complexities of movement, hormones, sleep, quality of food, and so much more. It also doesn't acknowledge the relationship between our thoughts and their impacts on our bodies. I can't pretend to understand this completely, but I can give you four reasons why working off dessert (or any other food for that matter) is counterproductive.

1. Working off dessert uses exercise as punishment

I have fond memories of my fourth-grade teacher, Mrs. Smith. Not only because she boldly sang our state song "Oklahoma" every morning, or because she smelled faintly of Mentholatum, but because she was fair. When one student got in trouble, she looked pointedly at that student and corrected him. If a consequence was necessary, it was directed to the offenders. Not once was I held back from recess because of something my classmate did.

In the same way, I shouldn't punish my body for a decision my brain made.

My body is made to move. She's also made to consume fuel—preferably foods from the earth—but she is designed to eat. My brain decides what to take from my hand and place it in my mouth. When my brain decides to indulge, it should not be my body's job to right that choice. Essentially, I am punishing my sweet body for a decision my brain made.

It's time we shift our thinking from exercise as being something we *have to do* to something we *get to do*. God gave us these incredible bodies that move forward, backward, side to side, and upside down. That only scratches the surface. Search for yoga or animal flow videos on Instagram or YouTube, and you'll see what I mean. The contortions some people can do are more complex than a full-term baby in the womb.

My body wants to move. She was designed to. Depending on the day, she prefers different activities. Sometimes she likes a full-out sprint, breathing so hard her abs are sore the next day. Other times she likes to lift heavy objects, and some days she prefers the gentle movement of yoga, mobility, and deep breathing.

What she doesn't like is being forced to work because of the choices my brain made. And she really doesn't like it when my brain has a negative attitude about it.

Exercise is not punishment; it's a gift. We were given one body, and while our souls may live forever in heaven, our body stays on this earth. I ought not to punish my body during its short time here.

2. Working off dessert is a joy-killer

A girlfriend of mine has a cherished family tradition: Sunday Sundae. Her family limits treats and sweets throughout the week, but on Sundays, her kids get to concoct the most outrageous dessert. Ice cream, sprinkles, chocolate syrup, and gummy bears (ew, but okay) all contribute to the creation. Watching her kids' eyes light up while they tell me about it proves how glorious it is. My friend joins on a smaller scale, most certainly without the gummy bears.

I imagine these Sunday nights are highly anticipated by her children. They plan what type of ice cream and toppings they'll choose. I picture closed-mouth smiles with a mouthful of cold bliss and perhaps a sprinkle stuck to the top of a lip.

It's a family tradition sure to be remembered.

Now take that beautiful moment and add an asterisk: *I have to work this off*. The intent of Sunday Sundae is to enjoy and indulge. On a deeper level, it's also meant to create fun memories and traditions as a family. Perhaps during this time the girls open up just a little more about their week or tell a story from English class that made them laugh so hard they snorted.

I have to work this off strips the laughter. The pleasure. The sacredness. We are taking something and adding shame to it and telling ourselves it's not worth it. And as we discussed above, it punishes our body for a choice our brain made.

It's also worth mentioning if *I have to work this off* is said out loud, what message is that giving those around us? My friend is fiercely protective of what her impressionable girls hear coming from her mouth. Like me, she's admitted to negative thoughts seeping in now and then. But she does her best to filter those thoughts before they become speech so her daughters hear less self-loathing and more self-acceptance coming from their own mother's mouth.

In her book *Think and Eat Yourself Smart*, Dr. Caroline Leaf teaches that the mindset behind a meal plays a commanding role in the process of human food-related health issues. According to research, our thought life controls 75–98 percent of illness including mental, physical, emotional, and behavioral issues.[1] Keep the joy in what you eat to keep healthy.

Maybe your family has a similar tradition to my friend, or maybe sometimes you just like to indulge. Do you visit a restaurant with your favorite dessert? Or perhaps your mother makes a German chocolate cake you can't resist.

How can we truly enjoy that German chocolate cake if the shame we have for it means we have to work it off? That has to be quite confusing for our brains. Shaming ourselves for the occasional indulgence steals joy from the moment.

3. Working off dessert makes for difficult math

Let's say you arrive at my house for Sunday Sundae (we now have them too). We pull out the Blue Bell Ice Cream and a pan of brownies for the special occasion. We all help ourselves to a two-inch square brownie. This isn't much, but it's the recommended serving on the back of the box. Then we add a one-half cup of vanilla ice cream. Again, not much. Between the brownie's 120 calories and the ice cream's 180, we have a small dessert totaling about 300 calories. If you were to order a dessert at a restaurant, however, that number may triple.

But let's say we just enjoyed our homemade dessert. The next morning we decide we need to work that off. Three hundred calories are about the equivalent of a three-mile walk or a forty-five-minute gym session. These numbers aren't hard science, as calorie burn varies based on a person's size and their exercise intensity, but are close enough.

Calories in, calories out, right? Now we have to take an extra forty-five minutes out of our day and exercise. And if you're wanting to be really precise, you'll need to do that on top of the time you already planned on exercising because, of course, you have to work off that dessert. If you generally do a forty-five-minute workout then add another forty-five minutes on to that, you're spending an hour and a half exercising. We'll talk later about why long, hard exercise sessions are not what's best for us. Besides, who has time for that anyway?

There's the physiological math too. When we show up at the gym the next morning, our joints may be a little inflamed from the sugar. What do you think working harder or longer will do? It certainly won't cause the inflammation to decrease. In fact, it does the opposite: it increases our risk of getting injured. I'm not saying we're going to experience a full ACL tear, but your knee may flare up. Or your back may feel tweaked.

This leads us back up to the first point: We have now punished our body for a decision our brain made.

Consider these other approaches: Either slightly decrease your caloric intake during the day, plan it as a treat day, or just enjoy it in the name of balanced eating and move on. Seriously. As my son would say, "It's just not that deep."

4. Working off dessert doesn't promote balance

For most of my early adult life, my health goal was simple: get a rocking body. I wanted abs worthy enough to sport a belly-button ring. I never got one. When I started learning about our food's health implications, I added a new goal: consume the highest-quality food that has the greatest return. Take blueberries, for example. At one point, Dr. Oz told me I should eat them. High in antioxidants, they can help my cells from aging and damage. I intentionally chose blueberries, envisioning glowing skin and happy cells bouncing around my body.

What started as a singular six-minute television segment turned into a fetish: blueberries in my shakes, muffins, and oatmeal. In the quest for optimum blueberry performance, I failed to recognize their other benefit: they taste delicious. I turned this God-given food into a means to healthy living, without recognition of the present enjoyment.

Today, while I'd still take a rocking body, my goal is different. Rather than sporting a belly-button ring, I choose the goal we discussed in the second chapter: *I want to take care of my body in a balanced and realistic way so I may do what I'm called to do today and in the future.*

Fast-forward to the time I accepted those belly-button-free abs. At some point, I recognized my need for balance. Yes, I needed to strengthen those ankles to achieve actual balance, but I also needed to have moments where I wasn't focused on food science. I needed to grab some blueberries simply because I like how they burst under slight pressure from my tongue. And I needed to stop shaming myself for enjoying foods that didn't have antioxidants and heart protection. I needed to enjoy an occasional dessert.

Enjoying dessert every now and then is realistic and balanced. Indulging every night impacts my sleep, inflames my joints, and makes focus difficult the next day. The sleep-deprived cycle continues when I look for quick hits in various forms to keep me awake: sugar, caffeine, and social media. My daily callings require more of me. Not once have I felt called to eat Oreos dunked in coffee while diving into the black hole of Twitter.

I'm also not interested in accumulating so many hours of exercise that my body breaks down. Working off dessert just adds to the hours, and I'm not interested. Forty-five minutes of exercise is joyful to me, believe it or not. Three hours is not—unless I'm hiking in the mountains with friends. Then I'll go until I drop. (But seeing how I live in the flatlands of Texas, this doesn't happen often.)

My goals may not be the same as yours. That's okay. But give them some thought if you haven't already. I'm betting an occasional dessert can fit nicely into your goals, and you don't even have to work it off.

The Simple Take:
Enjoy the occasional indulgence, and don't punish your
body for a decision your brain made.

A Little Bit of Chocolate Cake

Okay, this is actually a lot of chocolate cake. But we can't have a chapter that encourages you to enjoy dessert without it being chocolate. After all, I've been touting "Balanced healthy living with a lot of grace and a little chocolate" on my website since 2016.

This has become my go-to recipe when it's time to make a gluten-free decadent dessert. Top with your favorite frosting (a basic cream cheese/powdered sugar one works well), or just enjoy plain. It's that good.

The coconut oil adds a nice flavor. If you have a coconut allergy, use butter instead.

Ingredients

- 1 ½ cups semisweet chocolate chips
- ⅓ cup almond milk (or your preferred milk)
- 3 tbs. coconut oil
- 1 ½ cups almond flour/meal
- 1 tsp. baking soda
- ½ tsp. sea salt
- 1 tbs. sugar
- 2 large eggs, beaten
- 1 tsp. vanilla

Directions

Spray an 8x8 pan with nonstick spray. Preheat oven to 350 degrees.

Add the chocolate chips and milk to a saucepan. Heat over low heat, stirring frequently. When melted, add coconut oil and stir until melted. Turn off heat and set aside.

While chocolate chips are heating, mix the almond flour, baking soda, salt, and sugar in a medium bowl.

Whisk the eggs in a small bowl and add the vanilla.

Add the dry mix and egg mixture to the chocolate mixture. Fold everything in until mixed together.

Pour into prepared pan. Bake for 35 minutes or until a toothpick comes out clean.

When cooled, top with your favorite frosting.

CHAPTER SEVEN

It's all about the nutrients

Several years ago I found myself in Stillwater, Oklahoma, celebrating Oklahoma State University's Homecoming. My alma mater's homecoming consistently ranks as one of the best in the nation. One highlight is the House Decks created by the Greek system, which are the culmination of millions of colored tissues "pomped" into chicken wire to create visual storytelling. Pomping involves taking a four-by-four-inch square of tissue paper, wrapping it around the index finger, and shoving it through chicken wire in a preset pattern. It's mind-numbing and laborious, but the result is always an impressive House Deck. Several of my sorority sisters descended on this small college town to relive this experience and rejoice that we no longer had to pomp into the wee hours of the morning.

We met at my friend's house for dinner. She served an "Orange and Black Soup" to commemorate our university's colors. This hearty soup was a thick, savory blend of pumpkin puree, black beans, scallions, and ham. Alongside the soup, my friend served Caesar salad, crusty bread, and other delicious items. A cookbook holder held open the salad recipe. Always looking for inspiration, I began thumbing through it. It turned out to be a book with recipes rather than a cookbook.

"That's one of my favorites right now," explained my friend. Considering this same friend completed a fifty-two book challenge one year, that meant a lot. I looked at the front cover and was immediately smitten. *Bread and Wine* by Shauna Niequist had a picture of just that. Bread...I like bread. Wine...definitely like that. As described on Amazon:

> *"Bread and Wine" is a collection of essays about family relationships, friendships, and the meals that bring us together. It's a celebration of food shared, reminding readers of the joy found in a life around the table. It's about the ways God teaches and nourishes people as they nourish the people around them. It's about hunger,*

both physical and otherwise, and the connections between the two.[1]

Dinner at my friend's house that evening was exactly the kind of gathering around the table discussed in this beautiful book. Our twenty-year friendship has endured ups and downs. That night was filled with laughter and the joy of being together over a short twenty-four hours. Our conversations reminisced over those late-night pomping episodes, and we recalled collegiate escapades I probably shouldn't mention in a book my children might read one day.

Sitting around that kitchen island provided nourishment. Yes, my body was well fed from the soup and salad. But what felt more nourished was my soul. I love these friends dearly. My time with them always fills me with joy. Our annual girls trips don't always include soup and salad. They also include plenty of comfort food and spirits. But the nourishment these moments provide? Soul-filling, no matter what's on the menu.

Yes, food is fuel. It's something I stress in my nutrition lessons to teen summer-fitness clients. Food can make the difference between a good and bad workout, how well we recover after a gym session, how we feel at 3:00 p.m., and even how well we sleep. Just ask Shalane Flanagan, an American runner who won the New York Marathon after publishing a cookbook intended to fuel runners using whole-food recipes.

Whole foods (those in their natural state) provide quality fats, proteins, and carbs (including fiber) that are often lost in processing. Learning about nutrients helps me understand my body, what it needs, and what it may be telling me. My favorite fuel-based food is sweet potatoes, which seem to have a magical effect. They help me perform, recover, and sleep well. I choose vibrant salads for a variety of nutrients and fiber, which becomes more important with each passing year. Eggs provide me the perfect combination of protein and fat for satiety, and chickpeas give me protein and fiber without too many carbohydrates.

Science has provided more knowledge than ever on food's benefits:

- Want to increase your metabolism? Eat spicy foods. Capsaicin increases your metabolism.
- Muscle cramps? Grab some magnesium-rich foods like whole grains or nuts, which will help your muscles relax.
- Concerned about cancer? Dark-colored blueberries contain antioxidants that reduce DNA damage from everyday living.

We've been given so much information about the benefits of the foods we eat, we can forget to acknowledge one of the main benefits: fellowship.

Yes, God gave us food to fuel our bodies. He provided plants with many colors and a variety of animals from which to choose. He designed our bodies to need replenishment often. I get to choose from an assortment of foods and eat them three times a day! How glorious is that? Depending on what my body needs and is craving, I can choose a salad, sweet potato medallions with a small schmear of peanut butter, or grilled chicken. Compare that to my dog, Grace, who receives the *exact same* food twice a day, every day. How she is so excited for dinner time each day is a mystery. If someone told me today's menu plan was the same as yesterday and would be the same tomorrow, you can bet I would not joyfully bound over to the dinner table as she does to her bowl.

Yet here we are, with our abundant God-given foods. God told Adam, "*I give you every seed-bearing plant on the face of the whole earth and every tree that has fruit with seed in it. They will be yours for food*" (Gen. 1:29). God blessed Adam (and us) with a variety of ways to stop our growling stomachs.

Fast-forward to the Gospels, and we see Jesus enjoying those seed-bearing plants. He and the disciples break bread together, most notably in the Last Supper. While we don't know the specific foods that Jesus ate, based on the region's availability, we can deduce He consumed lentils, whole grains, fruits, vegetables, dates, nuts, and fish in accordance with Jewish dietary restrictions.

What we do have a record of is His time spent with His friends while eating. I believe this is not a coincidence. Yes, God specifically gave us food to fuel our bodies well. He also gave us people to enjoy meals with. Jesus used His time eating to serve and minister to others. He loved them, just as I love my college friends. They probably laughed just as we do. They shared stories. Perhaps they shared family or friendship struggles.

My mother likes to tell me the story of when I was a baby and she would grind up the "soup stew" she had prepared for her and my dad. Short on funds, it was easier and cheaper for her to blend carrots, onion, potatoes, green beans, celery, and cubed beef than to purchase baby food jars. She tells me I loved it. I still do. While I'm not a huge red meat eater, I still salivate over the thought of a warm pot of Mom's stew, simmering for hours. Mom once taught me the secret to tender stew was "simmer, simmer, simmer" for hours rather than quick cook. Often I arrived home from school on a cold February day to a stew simmering in preparation for dinner.

"Here, have a small cup. It's not completely ready, but it's more nourishing than a handful of crackers," she would say. Often I ladled a small amount into a teacup to appease her while rolling my eyes at the same time. Just as often I was glad I did. Through this small act, my mother was introducing me to the word "nourishment."

Nourish, as defined on Dictionary.com, is *"to sustain with food or nutriment; supply with what is necessary for life, health, and growth."*[2] Mom's stew certainly supplied "nutriment"—that is, food with plenty of nutrients. It also represented her love for me and the value she put on having quality dinners around the table every night.

Nourishment is a multidimensional word. Sometimes it's purely the nutrients within the food that promote life, health, and growth. Colorful salads with a variety of plant-based toppings certainly fall into this category. Other times nourishment encapsulates a dining experience. It spreads beyond the food we eat into the souls within us. A childhood friend of mine visited Houston on a work trip several years ago. She and I met for dinner. She shared stories of her daughter who possesses the same sass, laughter, and love of life as my friend. We caught up on each other's daily lives, marriages, and families of origin. We did all this over three hours and a chef's choice sushi-roll boat. While I'm sure that dinner didn't represent an ideal mix of fats, carbs (too much), and protein (too little), it nourished my soul. Lingering over our meal provided something no perfect mix of foods could provide. Dinner lifted my spirits and fostered our friendship. It left me on an emotional high for a few days. It bettered my life.

Proper nutrients have their place. I've found tracking my food periodically helps me ensure I'm eating the right amounts of protein, carbohydrates, and fats my specific body needs. When I exercise outdoors in the Houston summer, I'm intentional about eating high-potassium foods to replenish electrolytes lost in sweat, and I often supplement with a little magnesium to prevent nighttime muscle cramps. After my boys arrive home after a hard sports workout, I encourage them to eat well to replenish and repair their muscles (they might say I'm a little too neurotic about that).

But I've also discovered life, growth, and health is more than nutrients. It's experiences. Laughter. Stories. Memories. Bonding. Still, poor-quality foods, however soul-fulfilling they may be, won't keep my body functioning well for as long as possible. I can't dig into that cake nightly and expect to function well the next day. Meeting a friend every night for happy hour featuring a Sauvignon Blanc might be soul-filling, but it's sleep-stripping (thank you, wine hot flashes) and quite literally offers no nutrients.

Nevertheless, I'm willing to sacrifice perfect nutrients now and then for those soul-nourishing moments received in other ways. Sometimes I'm really lucky, and the two create a helix of intertwined quality food with a stellar conversation. I fiercely guard my Sunday-night family-dinner ritual. Between sports, church, and social events, we don't always sit around the table for weeknight dinners (though I do try hard to make that happen). Sunday nights, however, are nonnegotiable. This is when I practice the word "no" with myself and my children. No to dinner with friends. No to neighborhood ladies gatherings. No to school projects (you had all weekend to do that!). Yes to sitting down, often to grilled steelhead trout, asparagus, and roasted red potatoes. The menu is as predictable as the 6:30 sit-down time.

If I could handpick a positive memory my children have growing up, this would be one of them. We do a little calendar housekeeping, discussing schedules and appointments for the weeks. The rest of the time is often spent in deeper conversation: politics, fiscal policy, struggles with work, or debates the boys have had at school that roll over to the table. It may take twenty minutes to eat our food but an hour to enjoy the meal. And, of course, it ends with Sunday Sundae.

Each meal, we take turns thanking God for what He's given us. No matter who gives thanks, it almost always ends in something like "bless this food to the nourishment of our bodies."

Of course, there's another kind of nourishment. One that is filled not by foods and relationships but by He who provides us food and relationships: Jesus. I may not fully understand scripture, but this is what I do know: Even if every piece of my physical health is perfectly executed, I do not feel complete without Jesus. My morning time with Him and in God's word is critical for establishing my day's foundation.

This isn't to say I feel like I'm holier than thou. Quite the opposite. The more I learn, the more I realize how little I truly grasp the depth of God's love and grace.

God designed us to crave something more than we can receive here on earth. My body thirsts for water daily. Today I'm fancying something citrusy, maybe an orange and extra lemon squeeze in my water. I long for a workout if I miss several days. Nothing feels complete, though, without Jesus filling my soul. As John recounts, Jesus told His disciples, *"I am the bread of life. Whoever comes to me will never go hungry, and whoever believes in me will never be thirsty"* (John 6:35).

It's worth noting this came after two significant events earlier in the chapter. Jesus and the disciples were followed by several thousand people who were hoping to witness signs and miracles. Boy did they get one. Jesus took five small barley loves and two small fish offered up by a young boy, multiplied it, and fed five thousand men plus any women and children. The leftovers filled twelve baskets.

That evening, Jesus walked on the water during a strong storm. The following day, the crowd searched for Him. They realized even though He didn't board the boat with the disciples, He was on the other side of the lake. Again, we see hunger. This hunger was not one barley and fish could fill, but one of life.

If I don't start my day with Jesus (and coffee), I feel unsettled all day. My soul was meant to be filled by God the Father, Son, and Holy Spirit. Perhaps the most important meal of the day is that of the Bread of Life. I'm not wise enough to know how this all happens, but my experience confirms Jesus nourishes me more than any perfectly executed macro chart ever can.

God nourishes our bodies in so many ways. Some through the foods He's given us. Some through our relationships and Orange and Black Soup. Some with memories in the making, whether it's dinner rituals or soup stew. But they all provide life, health, and growth. Additionally, He designed our soul to be nourished by Him alone, which also provides life, health, and growth. And that, my friends, is true nourishment.

The Simple Take:
Nutrients have their place, but so does the nourishment provided by enjoying a meal with friends and family...
even if it's not perfectly balanced.

Orange and Black Soup
(adapted from Epicurious.com)

Fair warning: The title of this soup describes the colors that go into it, not the end result. However, the flavors come together nicely for a robust soup. Don't skip the sherry and rice vinegar — they add a unique element.

Ingredients

- Three 15-oz. cans black beans, rinsed and drained
- 1 can petite diced tomatoes
- 2 tbs. butter
- 1 onion, chopped
- 1 shallot, finely chopped
- 3 cloves garlic, minced
- 1 tbs. ground cumin
- 1 tsp. salt
- ½ tsp. fresh ground pepper
- 4 cups broth (beef for more robust flavor, chicken for more mild)
- One 15-oz can pumpkin puree (not pie filling)
- ½ cup sherry cooking wine
- 1 lb. cooked ham, diced
- 3 tbs. rice wine vinegar
- Serve with crusty bread (better yet, a bread bowl!)

Directions

Use a food processor or immersion blender in a glass bowl to coarsely blend the black beans and tomatoes. Add a little water or extra broth if necessary to help blend.

In a 6-quart pot, sauté onion, shallot, and garlic in butter with the spices: cumin, salt, and pepper.

Stir in bean and tomato puree, broth, pumpkin puree, and sherry cooking wine. Simmer uncovered for 25 minutes. Add in diced ham and rice vinegar just before serving. Add additional salt and pepper if desired (remember, ham has high sodium, so do this after you add the ham).

This recipe does serve a crowd. My favorite trick is to make the full batch then freeze in individual portions for easy meals later.

CHAPTER EIGHT

Carbs are the enemy

Several years ago, a friend shared an unusual way her father healed from a Lou Gehrig's (ALS) diagnosis. The treatment wasn't scientifically and research-backed, so I don't think this book is an appropriate place to share what it was. But, as she explained more, she told me how her father gave up carbs as well. He felt better than ever and had more life and mobility than he had in years.

"All carbs?" I asked. "Like he doesn't even have fruit?"

"Oh, he has fruit," she clarified. "But he doesn't eat any bread or pasta or anything."

I have an annoying habit of correcting people. I'm aware of this. But this time I kept my mouth shut and decided not to remind her that her dad, indeed, did consume carbs if he ate fruits and vegetables.

Carbohydrates, one of the three food macronutrients (along with protein and fat), get a bad rap. Some of this is with good reason: our standard American diet is heavy on refined grains (like white bread and white rice) and various forms of fried potatoes and corn. In general, we consume too many of these ...way too many.

But think about the Garden of Eden. What do you think was harvested there? We know apples, which doesn't make a great argument at the moment. Deuteronomy 8:7-8 gives us some more insight into what our biblical ancestors consumed:

> *For the Lord your God is bringing you into a good land, a land of brooks of water, of fountains and springs, flowing forth in valleys and hills; a land of wheat and barley, of vines and fig trees and pomegranates, a land of olive oil and honey.*

Wheat, barley, figs, pomegranates, olive oil, honey. Sounds delicious. Except for the olive oil, all of these contain carbohydrates.

What are carbohydrates, and what do they do?

Carbohydrates' primary role is to provide energy to the body. Carbs are naturally occurring sugars, starches, and fiber in your food. You'll find these in fruits, grains, vegetables, and milk. (Trick: If an ingredient ends in "-ose," it's a sugary carb.) They are the first line of ingestion over fats and protein and are easily absorbed into the bloodstream. If you grew up adoring the movie *Steel Magnolias*, this is why Julia Roberts's character, Shelby, was given orange juice when diabetes caused her blood sugar to drastically drop. The high sugar in orange juice could easily be uploaded into the blood system to help stabilize her blood sugar.

Another forgotten and neglected element of carbohydrates is fiber. Fiber helps empty the stomach, reduces your risk for cardiovascular disease, reduces potential blood-sugar spikes, and improves the absorption of foods. Fiber is only found in carbohydrates and plays a vital role in how quickly something is digested and used as energy. The more fiber a food has, the longer it takes to digest. This is a good thing as it helps you to feel fuller longer and regulates your blood sugar better. And of course, it promotes bowel movement and intestinal health. If you've ever tried or led a low-carb diet, you may have discovered your, *ahem*, bathroom time was less efficient.

Sugars: Yay or nay?

There's a lot of confusion out there about sugar. That's understandable. Is it good? Is it bad? Is some okay? What's not okay? First, my philosophy is there are no "good" and "bad" foods. But there are foods that offer more value than others. Sugar is a great example of this. Sugar in any form, whether it's a white cube or a ripe banana, is quickly digested and pushed into the bloodstream. The difference is what comes along for the ride. That white cube—or, more practically speaking, the Sprite and Sour Patch Kids gummy candy that my kids love—carries nothing else of value. While I don't believe every single food we consume needs to have quality nutrients (as we talked about in the last chapter), most should. Ripe bananas contain fiber, potassium, vitamin B6, vitamin C, magnesium, copper, and manganese. Sour Patch Kids, on the other hand, have a bunch of fake food coloring.

Your body treats sugar the same way regardless of what food it came in. It's uploaded into the bloodstream and taken to your muscles and liver (more on this below). However, what comes along with sugar makes a huge difference in how everything else functions.

Added sugar is what we want to avoid. This is the valueless sugar that doesn't contain nutrients. The American Heart Association recommends limiting *added* sugar to six added teaspoons per day.[1] (Hey, look at that. Even the AHA allows for balance.) Let's quantify what six added teaspoons are. One teaspoon contains four grams of sugar, and one gram of sugar equals four calories, so for six teaspoons, that would be ninety-six calories. You want to keep that added sugar to around one hundred calories a day. Keep in mind food manufacturers get sneaky with the added sugar, so check your labels.

How does our carb consumption relate to our everyday life?

As I mentioned, carbohydrates provide energy to the body. Think of them as fuel for all your organs, muscles, and tissues. This is also a helpful analogy when determining what kind of carbs to ingest. Your body is like a Lamborghini, and it functions best on premium fuel. When we choose a lower-grade fuel, we don't run optimally.

When you consume carbohydrates, your body digests them into glucose and takes it to several areas.

Bloodstream

Your blood holds a small amount of glucose in the event you need a short, quick burst of energy for a few seconds. The rest is transported elsewhere.

Liver

The liver holds a limited amount of glycogen (the word for stored glucose). This glycogen provides energy in a more constant state and is released to keep your blood sugar stable in between meals.

Muscles

Glycogen in your muscles is used solely by your muscles. Think of it as a gift to your muscles with an "especially for you" tag on it. This is what your muscles tap into during long periods of exercise. The general rule of thumb is you run out of glycogen in your muscles after about forty-five minutes, which is why you'll see long-distance athletes consuming a sport gel or gummy after about an hour. The muscles are out of energy, and that quick fix of sugar helps provide the necessary energy to sustain movement.

Brain

One organ that relies on carbohydrates is the brain. Even though the brain accounts for just about 2 percent of our total body weight, the brain uses about 20 percent of glucose-derived energy, making it the main consumer of glucose in the body.[2] Glucose is what your body creates, with the help of insulin, as it breaks down the food in the stomach. Glucose-derived energy is what carbohydrates turn into if they aren't already in their simplest state, like pure sugar. Once I tried a low-carb diet. Walking through a hardware aisle in Lowe's, I suddenly doubled over with a splitting headache. It came on hard and fast, pleading for a banana. My brain missed those carbohydrates.

Adipose tissue

Once everything gets what it needs, glucose is stored for future use. Your body doesn't know when it might need it again, so it holds onto it. Some adipose is good; in fact, for women in their forties, the recommended amount is 23-25 percent of their total weight.[3] Adipose is a word you'll hear me using throughout this book. It's the formal word for body fat. Unfortunately, many of us have a complicated relationship with the term body fat, so I use adipose more often than not.

Why do carbs get a bad rap? A Disney story starring refined and unrefined carbs.

Let's answer this question with a story of the three Tremaine sisters from the classic Disney story *Cinderella*. To refresh your memory, the sisters' names are Anastasia, Drizella, and, of course, Cinderella.

Anastasia and Drizella are also known as the evil stepsisters. They are self-absorbed, have no regard for others, and offer no value. They junk up the house and don't do anything to contribute to it. Their mood shifts from energetic to cranky in a heartbeat.

Refined carbohydrates, like white sugar and white flour, are the evil stepsisters. They are given, and some might argue deserve, a bad rap because they add no value. They spike our blood sugar and then come crashing down, just like the stepsisters' moods. Refined carbs are foods created in a manufacturing plant rather than a plant from the ground.

Not only do they not provide the nutrients our body needs to function well, but they also cause inflammation. It's like they are walking through the house, dropping their candy bar wrappers and potato chip bags, creating more clutter for sweet Cinderella to pick up. Cinderella can't focus on the things she loves to do because she's picking up Milky Way wrappers all day.

Cinderella, on the other hand, is hard-working, diligent, and positive. Productive carbs, or Cinderella carbs, add value. They carry nutrients to your blood and provide fiber. Cinderella carbs are foods that are plants, not foods made in one. These are the fruits, vegetables, and whole grains we discussed earlier.

The right kind of carbohydrates makes all the difference in the world. As I mentioned earlier, one of my favorite carbohydrates is sweet potatoes. When I'm running, I notice a huge difference in my performance and how I feel when I've been enjoying sweet potatoes. Strangely enough, they also help me sleep. Sweet potatoes are great sources of fiber, antioxidants, and vitamins.

The problem with stepsister carbs is they are easier to consume, leading to us eating more of them than we need. When foods are processed and refined, they are often stripped of fiber and general bulk that slows the eating process down. For example, a medium banana contains about 100 calories. If one bunch has six bananas, that's 600 calories. Oreos, on the other hand, are highly refined and offer little nutritional value. Two Oreos hold 140 calories. If you grabbed a package of Oreos, you'd find twelve of them lined up neatly in three rows. It's pretty easy to plow through one row without much thought. This row contains 840 calories. Eating an entire bunch of six bananas, however, seems daunting.

While I don't like to get too focused on the calories of items (I spent too much of my younger years doing this and consider myself a recovering calorie counter), I think it's helpful to understand the value of our foods. Those stepsister carbs are sneaky, and you can easily eat way more than you intended.

Fruit is an excellent source of carbohydrates. To quote one of my friends: "Anybody who doesn't believe in God has never had watermelon."

She has a point. Fresh, ripe watermelon explodes in your mouth and ignites your taste buds. It also provides a host of nutritional benefits, including offering hydration, fiber, electrolytes, and the antioxidant lycopene. Only God could combine such flavor and nutrients in one food. Yet some avoid this amazing fruit because of its carb and sugar content.

That doesn't mean our diet should consist solely of watermelon or any other food He gave us, for that matter. The good news is God didn't give us only one food. He gave us a huge variety, each to nourish our body and to be enjoyed.

Carbs are not the enemy. Carbs are a necessary part of a balanced diet. Aim to choose Cinderella carbs: fruits, whole grains, and vegetables, rather than evil-stepsister refined carbs. How much should you have? Tune in to the next chapter for a recommended range.

I recognize our bodies thrive on and require different amounts of carbohydrates. Type 1 diabetics must watch their intake to control their blood sugar. Perhaps the data in this chapter does not apply to them. Likewise, research has indicated a ketogenic diet can be beneficial in managing epilepsy.[4] If that's you, stick with what's best for your body, not the general science I'm providing here.

Speaking of the ketogenic diet, I recognize our body can convert fat to energy. The ketogenic diet involves consuming a large percentage of calories from fat, a moderate percentage of protein, and very little carbohydrates. This combination leads to nutritional ketosis. Nutritional ketosis occurs when the body breaks down fat in the absence of carbohydrates. The body can now use these ketones as a fuel source to generate energy instead of energy from carbohydrates.[5]

If that program works for you, then go for it. I hear prominent, educated influencers share how well it makes them feel. I certainly know better than to shame them or anyone who chooses to eat a ketogenic diet. But as for me and my body, I will happily ingest carbs.

Overall, I think we fail to appreciate all that God has given us when we swear off carbs (except for those certain medical conditions). But for the rest of us, I think it's time we stop thinking of carbohydrates as bad for us and start thinking of them as resources for our body. If Cinderella's evil stepsisters had helped her with the housework rather than making it worse, perhaps the story would have ended differently. Instead of the Fairy Godmother saving the day by allowing Cinderella to go to the ball, perhaps she would have figured out what makes her feel mentally and physically strong. We could have seen Cinderella morph into Wonder Woman! Adding those good carbohydrates can help you feel mentally and physically strong as well. Eat the right amount of foods God gave us to go out there and conquer the world.

The Simple Take:
Carbohydrates are a beneficial part of the food God gave us. Just try to consume more of the natural plants He provides rather than those created in a manufacturing plant.

Cinderella Baked Oats

For this recipe, I wanted to provide a nutrient-rich carb the whole family will love with easy prep and cleanup. This baked oatmeal is full of Cinderella carbs—the ones that add value and benefit to our daily living.

Nutritional Value

- **Rolled oats.** Fiber, lowers blood-sugar levels, promotes healthy gut bacteria, protein (½-cup serving offers 6g), iron
- **Bananas.** Potassium, fiber, vitamin B6
- **Apples.** Vitamin C, fiber (including pectin, a type of fiber that promotes gut health)
- **Carrots.** Vitamin A, vitamin K
- **Pumpkin.** Vitamin C, vitamin A, fiber
- **Dark chocolate.** Types with 70 percent or more provide antioxidants, iron, and magnesium

Just like with our workouts, customize this recipe to your liking.

Ingredient notes:

- **Sweetener.** I prefer local, raw honey as I try to consume a little each day to help manage allergies. You may also use maple syrup or sugar.
- **Apples.** You may peel the apple before dicing. I leave the skin on, as this is where much of the fiber is held. The smaller you dice the apple, the less you'll notice the skin.
- **Carrots.** Use julienned or matchstick carrots and chop to save time instead of grating. Alternatively, you can take baby carrots and finely chop them.

Ingredients

- 4 cups rolled (old-fashioned) oats
- 1 tsp. baking powder
- 2 tsp. cinnamon
- ¼ tsp. salt
- ¼ cup honey
- ¼ cup unsalted butter, melted and slightly cooled
- 2 ripe medium bananas, mashed
- 1 large egg
- ¾ cup pumpkin puree
- 1 cup your choice milk
- 1 Granny Smith apple, diced
- 1 cup grated carrots (about 1.5–2 carrots)
- 3 oz. 70 percent dark chocolate bar, chopped
- 1 cup walnuts, chopped (optional)

Directions

Preheat the oven to 350 degrees. Spray a 13x9 baking pan with nonstick spray.

In a medium bowl, mix oats, baking powder, cinnamon, and salt. Set aside.

In a separate bowl, combine mashed bananas, egg, honey, pumpkin puree, and milk. Then add melted butter (this prevents the heated butter from slightly cooking the egg).

Combine the dry ingredients with wet ingredients. Add in apple, carrots, chocolate, and walnuts. Pour and pat into baking pan. Bake for 35 minutes. Let cool 5 minutes before serving.

Store in the refrigerator or freezer, not on the counter. I cut the pan into squares and put half into the fridge for the week. The other half I individually wrap in plastic wrap and freeze for later. My recipe testers and I learned the hard way that if you leave the bars on the counter, they get moldy. Ew.

CHAPTER NINE

There's one best diet

For years, my husband and I prepared our own taxes. Thankfully, there were many resources online where we could enter our income, deductions, and everything else and submit it all to Uncle Sam. As our finances became more complicated, we decided we needed more expertise than what we had, so we enlisted the help of a CPA.

You will hear me speaking throughout this book of the importance of hiring a Certified Personal Trainer if you choose to get professional help with your fitness. I taught group fitness classes as a certified group fitness instructor for thirteen years before taking the next step and getting my personal trainer certification. I admit I walked into the personal trainer education thinking I knew everything. Boy, was I wrong. In fact, much of my passion of health education came through those six months I spent studying. I learned more than I expected and have implemented that into both training my clients and myself.

I am also a certified nutrition coach. What does that mean? It means I spent several months learning the basic nutritional science about food and how it relates to our body. Quite honestly, the only reason I pursued this certification is to provide authority when I give short nutrition lessons to my teen clients. At the end of my summer teen classes, I tell them to drink their water and eat real foods, and I educate them on the difference between carbs, fats, and proteins. I wanted to have some credibility behind my name before I taught impressionable young women whom were entrusted to me by their parents.

I've seen some grumbling among registered dietitians that personal trainers and nutrition coaches provide too much nutrition guidance outside of their expertise. This is fair. Just like my CPA knows more about taxes than I do, a registered dietitian knows more than I do about the science of food.

Despite my philosophy on this, I still receive questions often about which is the best diet. That's fair as well. We can't enter a new year without some new form of eating being introduced ever so conveniently in December.

Let's talk about a few ways we can evaluate what is, indeed, the best diet. And by diet, I mean an eating or nutrition program. The word "diet" conjures up restriction and hangry behavior, so I choose to use more-positive language.

Here are some questions to ask to determine what nutrition program is best for you.

Does it include the basic tenants of food?

We can't get out of the first book of the Bible without witnessing God's provision: "*I give you every seed-bearing plant on the face of the whole earth and every tree that has fruit with seed in it. They will be yours for food*" (Gen. 1:29). Later, He includes animals. "*Everything that lives and moves about will be food for you. Just as I gave you the green plants, I now give you everything*" (Gen. 9:3).

Somewhere along the way, we've lost the beauty of God's abundance and forgotten that all of these foods provide value. Let's quickly talk about these.

All food contains at least one of three elements, also called macronutrients: fats, carbohydrates, and protein. Some, like chicken breast, may have mostly protein, a little fat, and no carbohydrates. Others, like strawberries, are mostly carbohydrates.

Here's a quick lesson on these three macronutrients:

- *Carbohydrates.* Carbohydrates, as we just discussed, provide energy to your muscles and brain. Carbs are found in fruit, vegetables, and grains.

- *Proteins.* Proteins are multifunctional. They make muscles and tissues, play a role in carrying oxygen throughout the body, repair damaged muscles from working out, and help produce antibodies that protect your immune system. You'll find high protein in meat, fish, eggs, and dairy. It's also present in beans and legumes.

- *Fats.* Fats help your body absorb certain vitamins and gives you energy. "Good fats," formally known as mono- or poly-unsaturated fats, may help heart health by improving cholesterol levels. "Bad fats," or saturated and trans fats, raise the low-density lipoprotein (LDL) cholesterol, which can increase your risk of heart disease. Stick with those unsaturated fats, like those founds in olives, nuts, and fatty fish, as much as possible.

You need all three of these to thrive. Even the ketogenic diet, which heavily focuses on healthy fats, recommends that 5–10 percent of daily calories come from carbs.

The National Academy of Medicine[1] reports the acceptable distribution range as:

- 45–65 percent of calories from carbs
- 10–35 percent of calories from proteins
- 20–35 percent of calories from fats

Before you step into any program, make sure it encompasses the variety of foods God provided. They are there for a reason.

What is realistic?

Suppose we learned today that science has discovered the very best way to eat is by consuming steak, mashed potatoes, and gravy. Several members of my household would be thrilled beyond measure and might be considered some of the healthiest people in the world. I, however, would not. I enjoy red meat on occasion, but in general it tears up my stomach and wakes me up in the middle of the night.

Mashed potatoes are fine if they are prepared simply but not with a bunch of butter and milk.

Eating steak everyday would not be realistic for me. I just couldn't get excited to pull out a sharp knife and eat it on a regular basis. You may have heard about benefits from various diets: paleo, ketogenic, gluten-free, DASH, Mediterranean. All have varying forms of science-backed positive aspects. As I write, the Mediterranean diet is being hailed as the healthiest. By the time this book is released, we may have something else holding that title.

What is the most realistic way for you to eat on a daily basis? What can you actually adhere to most of the time? If you are excited about a keto plan but eat out regularly, this may be more challenging. Restaurants often use sugars and carbs to enhance their meals. And I don't know about you, but I have a hard time passing on the chip basket at Mexican restaurants. If something only works under certain circumstances with no variation allowed for real life, perhaps this is not realistic where are you on a long-term basis. Which leads me to...

What is sustainable?

There's a big difference between trying something for a period of time and deciding this is your new normal. I've seen friends complete thirty-day or six-week programs successfully. Sometimes these are used as a reset after a season of not taking care of their nutrition as well as they would like. Sometimes it's just to try something new and see what their body responds to. Or perhaps they are just being supportive of a loved one who wants to try it. All of these I applaud. I certainly don't mean to dissuade you from trying any specific eating program. In fact, I encourage you to try anything you are interested in that has research-based positive aspects. I've done this before under the title of experimentation.

But when you decide you want to participate in an eating plan long-term, ask yourself if you can actually do it long-term. We all get excited the first few days and weeks of trying something new. It seems like something we can sustain forever. But then life sets in, and our wherewithal decreases.

Several years ago, I enlisted the help of a registered dietitian as I prepared for a sprint triathlon. I really wanted to see how well I could perform if I combined arduous training and solid nutrition. Each week I submitted a food log and we reviewed it. One of the items we discussed was my bean dip. I've heard some of my fellow Texans call this Cowboy Caviar. It's basically a combination of various beans, vegetables, and herbs. I also throw in a little mango for a sweet kick. My husband and I enjoy this as a meal during the summer and eat it with Tostitos Scoops chips. And yes, I get the regular kind, not baked. I have nothing against baked chips, but I prefer the taste and simpler ingredients of the regular ones.

My dietitian applauded the bean dip but recommended I eat it over a bed of greens. Yes, this is a solid piece of nutrition advice. Swapping out chips for salad is rarely a bad idea. I recommend it. However, after a couple times of that variation, I realized I really missed the chips. I missed the crunch and I missed sharing the bowl with my husband. This is a microexample of sustainability. It suited me well for that season. I placed second in my race. But I now eat chips with my bean dip because the greens weren't sustainable (plus I get plenty of my greens elsewhere in my diet, thank you very much).

If you're looking at an eating program and think it might be for you, give it a shot. But if it's something you can't do for the long run, consider it an experiment, not a program. There is nothing wrong with experiments. And there is nothing wrong with deciding that a diet or eating program is not sustainable for you. Take the time to figure out a plan you can do for the long haul. The following are some questions to consider when choosing an eating program or plan:

- How much time does it take to prepare and plan your meals? Do you have that amount of time?

- Who will eat this way? If you have to create a completely different menu for you than the rest of your family, are you willing to do that?

- Consider what message the plan/program may send your people. Will they perceive what you are doing as admirable, or might they think, "If this is what healthy is, I'm not interested?"

- Does this plan/program fit into my lifestyle?

- Six months from now, how will I feel about this plan/program?

To be clear, I'm not advocating you throw all plans out the window in the name of it not being realistic and sustainable. Give whatever you're doing a fair shot. There's no firm guidance on this, but I recommend at least three to four weeks. Also remember you don't have to go all in at once. Perhaps you need to baby step your way into a program that looks interesting, more gradually incorporating it into your life.

Is it grounded in science and evidence-based research?

In the past election cycle, my kids and I had a lot of conversations about where they got their political news. It's no secret that social media uses algorithms to determine what we see and we tend to get the same types of content fed to us whether we realize it or not. I counseled my boys to evaluate the source of their political information and to make sure that information came from a reputable news company. We reviewed infographics on how certain news sources lean, and I encouraged them to read from sources on the right, left, and middle. I also advised them to fact-check anything that seemed strange. My friend Barbara, who is a journalist, taught me that if a headline invoked emotion, there is a strong possibility the article was slanted.

YOUR WORTHY BODY

So too can our nutrition information be. We may click on a link our friend shares or do a little research, and all of a sudden we are inundated with posts about that type of eating. Unfortunately, those posts are not as accurate as they would like us to believe they are. And if the claims they make look too good to be true, they probably are.

The best nutrition programs are those backed with science and evidence-based research. Science uses a specific unbiased process to obtain knowledge. (Remember the scientific method we learned in eighth grade? Yep, that's the one.) This process includes formulating explanations and testing them with experiments and data. It's not merely based on something we read on the internet or something a friend told you worked well. Evidence-based research takes that science, makes field observations, and takes into consideration individual client needs and preferences. Educate yourself about what the programs claim, especially if it seems extreme. You can do this through academic textbooks, university public health websites, the Academy of Nutrition and Dietetics website (eatright.org), and US government and international health websites.

Take the time to learn about the style and type of food program you are interested in. Even the intuitive-eating method, which focuses on the personal process of honoring your health and listening and responding to the direct messages of your body in order to meet your physical and psychological needs,[2] is evidence-based.

What makes you feel the best?

For lunch today, I had a kale salad with buckwheat and lemon miso dressing topped with pepitas. On the side, I enjoyed some sweet potato fries cooked in the air fryer. Yesterday I had a breakfast burrito from a fast-food chain that included a white flour tortilla, breaded chicken nuggets, cheese, and hash browns. Both of these meals are delicious. Only one, however, left me feeling clearheaded and that

126

perfect combination of satisfied yet still light. I think you can figure out which one was which. And while I don't advocate eating fast food for every meal, I do I think we need to give ourselves the grace to do so every now and then.

But when I pay attention to the foods I eat and how I feel as a result of that, I have incentive to keep going back to the ones that reward me. Sure, that breakfast burrito was rewarding in the moment. However, I felt pretty crummy the rest of the afternoon.

The best nutrition program is the one that makes you feel energetic, clearheaded, and able to do what you are called to do for the rest of the day. You won't hear me advocating for one over the other. Some of us need the freedom to make individual decisions based on our daily needs (hand raised). Others thrive on a strict, regimented program. For years I tsk-tsked this approach until I realized that just because it wasn't best for me didn't mean it wasn't best for somebody else.

If you don't know where to start or who to trust, use this litmus test: Does the plan recommend eating real food? Can you hold the food item in your hand and determine where it came from? An animal? The ground? A tree? You will receive more nutrients and benefits from foods with easily recognizable sources. Some people call this whole-food nutrition, or single-ingredient foods. Basically, did God give this to us to eat? If so, dig in. If not, enjoy sparingly. Just like my chocolate.

The Simple Take:
The best diet is the one that is realistic and sustainable, advocates God-given foods, and makes you feel the best.

Texas Caviar

I make this recipe on a Friday night as a meal for my husband, and we have plenty of leftovers for the rest of the weekend. I've provided the base, but customize to your liking:

Ingredients

- 1 can black-eyed peas, rinsed and drained
- 1 can black beans, rinsed and drained
- 1 can corn, rinsed and drained
- 1 red pepper, chopped
- 1 yellow pepper, chopped
- 1 jalapeño pepper, seeds removed, chopped
- 2–4 Roma tomatoes, seeded and chopped
- 1 mango, chopped
- Handful of cilantro, chopped
- ½ cup dressing of choice, more if desired

Mix it up

- Add red onion.
- Add avocado (best to add right before eating).
- Substitute basil and/or mint instead of cilantro.
- Add a spice like cumin or chili powder.

Directions

Combine all ingredients in a bowl. Add in desired dressing. Most of the time I'm lazy and simply use a purchased lite Italian dressing. Other times I'm more energetic and do an equal part olive oil and lime juice (⅓ cup each) with a tablespoon or two of honey. Start with ½ cup or so of dressing; taste and add more if desired. You can always add more but can't take it out!

Enjoy with tortilla chips or a bed of greens (even if you're not training for a triathlon).

CHAPTER TEN

Jump in and get 'er done

*A*s a fitness professional, I must achieve hours of education every two years to maintain my certification. In 2016, I enrolled myself in an all-day program that offered a new format I could bring back to my clients and class participants.

At some point during the day, our master trainer mentioned the importance of performing push-ups correctly. "Oh, I got this," I thought. "He may be a master trainer, but I'm a master push-upper." (No, there's no certification for this. I was just that confident.) He went through each step, educating us about each one. He went on: "Otherwise, you'll end up overtraining your pectorals and will find you have upper-crossed syndrome, which causes your shoulders to cave in even when you stand up straight." He looked directly at me. "Some of you already exhibit the signs of this."

Oof.

He was right. As I learned all the intricacies that go into executing a proper plank (the foundation of a push-up), I realized I had, in fact, been doing my push-ups wrong my entire life. And my slightly caved-in shoulders were proof.

We have a mindset that the meat of the workout is the most important part and that when we do this main section, we need to pay more attention to *what* we are doing than *how*. If you need proof, do a quick search on Pinterest for "exercise." A brief scroll of the pins shows plenty of workouts; many of them look solid, but few include any mention of a warm-up, cooldown, or form. This book offers you applicable resources at the end of each chapter, many of which are ways to move your body by working out. Before we get into those, I want to give you some basic guidelines.

Warm-up

The purpose of the warm-up is to prepare your body for physical activity. You'll want to mimic the movements you plan on doing. For example, before a run, you might walk. If you are power walking, start off slower. If you're doing a lower-body workout, then do some lower-body movements like squats and lunges (more on this as a stretching mechanism in a minute). In general, a warm-up should last five to ten minutes. The newer you are to formal exercise, the longer you should warm up.

You also need to prepare your cardiorespiratory system: your heart and lungs. At rest, our body pumps about five liters of blood per minute. Your heart delivers oxygenated blood to your muscles and the rest of your body at a steady rate. Think of traffic along a high-way that's moving smoothly, with cars entering and exiting with ease and everybody going about the same speed. The volume is consistent. Take that same highway and thrust four times as many cars on an on-ramp all at the same time. This is like your heart pumping more blood but your lungs not being up to speed. Your lungs take the deoxygenated blood that's moved through your body and reoxygenate it with the air you're breathing. Eventually, all the cars settle in and move along well, but it was pretty congested for a while.

So, too, do your heart and lungs need to ramp up together. When you warm up, you are taking your heart from pumping five liters of blood per minute to twenty to forty. Part of the warm-up is designed to give it time to do this. If you're a runner, you know that the first mile is always the hardest. Always. Walking out the door and im-mediately running will make you wonder how you're going to get through the next few miles. (Which gives credit to the recommen-dation of walking before running.) Then, as if by magic, everything feels better after a mile or so.

This gap time from beginning the workout to feeling in a rhythm is the time your heart and lungs are getting established. When I taught indoor cycling classes, I always felt a little sheepish being out of breath so early on. Thirty minutes in, I could verbalize the cues without feeling so winded. This, too, was simply the gap.

When we fail to give ourselves time to warm up, our heart and lungs have a hard time adapting. And our muscles? That leads to...

Stretching

When I was in high school, my dance team would break into several small groups to prepare for our practice. When I led my group, I typically would start by having us take our legs wide and fold our upper body over. We would stay there a bit, then move our torso to the right and hold, and the same on our left. We moved through the lower body to prepare our legs for kicking as high as possible, holding each stretch for long periods of time.

No, no, no.

Yes, stretching is good. Don't neglect that. But that approach right before a workout could have injured me. I'll explain why in a minute.

"So, Amy, how *am* I supposed to stretch?" I'm glad you asked.

First, start by moving your body. You can do this with a cardiovascular movement, like walking or biking. You can also mimic the moves you'll be doing later but at a lower intensity. Squat with no weights, do push-ups on your knees or not as deep, or use light weights.

Then, employ one of these techniques.

Self-myofascial release (SMR)

SMR, otherwise known as foam rolling, involves moving your muscles along a dense roller to release dense muscle fibers, or knots. This is particularly helpful for those really tight areas, as it helps release any "knots" in your connective tissue and muscles. SMR can also help your connective tissue. If you find your joints consistently sounding like Rice Krispies (snap, crackle, pop), foam rolling may help release tight connective tissue that contributes to this. Rather than going into depth here on how to foam roll, I've created a video in the free resource guide as a supplement to Chapter 15.

Dynamic stretching

This type of stretch uses continual movement and momentum to move the joint through a full range of motion. For example, if you stand on one foot and begin moving the other foot forward and back like a pendulum, this is dynamic stretching. The key is to start easy and increase that range of motion as the muscles warm up. In the pendulum example, your kick may start just a foot off the ground, but you will slowly increase the height as your muscles get acclimated. Dynamic stretching is what we do when we squat, lunge, reach, and push our way through the beginning of a workout. Most of my warm-ups utilize dynamic stretching.

Active stretching

The first time I tried active stretching I was blown away. The science behind it is called reciprocal inhibition, which is contracting one muscle while relaxing the opposing muscle. Doing this actually helps stretch the opposing muscle even more. For example, lie on your back with straight legs. Elevate one leg as high as you are comfortable. Grab your calf or hamstring (the back of your leg), and pull it toward your chest while pressing your leg against your hands. Hold for one or two seconds, and release. Do this five to ten times, and you'll notice you may be able to draw that straight leg much closer to your chest. This is a great one to have some help with, so if you have a partner you trust, they can help you deepen that press and subsequent stretch. *Please* make sure this partner will listen to your cues to how far to take the foot. The last thing we need is someone who decides your leg needs to go down farther than your body is ready for and ends up injuring you.

Static stretching

Chances are when the word "stretch" comes to mind, this type of stretching is what you envision. This is what my dance team groups did. Static stretching involves taking a muscle to the point of tension and holding it for thirty seconds or more. When you hold that stretch (tension) for thirty seconds, it creates release by the Golgi tendon organ. This organ is located at the end of your muscle and exists to protect your muscles from lengthening, or stretching, too far. Basically, holding that point of tension for thirty seconds tells the Golgi tendon organ that your muscles are safe and can be lengthened a little further. Performing static stretching right before exercising may lead your muscles to falsely assume they can extend farther than they can. In the case of my dance team, I could have kicked too high and strained my muscle. If you're wanting to increase your flexibility, this is the approach to take, but do it *after* a workout. Current science tells us that static stretching may decrease strength and power, so it's best you save your static stretches for your postworkout.[1]

Which stretch to use? It depends. (You'll see this ambiguity often in this book. That's because I want to empower you to figure out what is best for you in various situations.) How your body is feeling, how sore you are, and your goals for the workout all influence this decision. Personally, I don't think you can go wrong with dynamic stretching and some foam rolling if you're extra sore or tight.

Form

I am the most grace-giving trainer I can be, except in one area: form. Sometimes I wonder if my new clients are rolling their eyes in their heads as I tweak their positions. As we get older, we should be even more concerned about proper form as improper positioning can cause injury.

It's difficult to cover all aspects of form in one section of one chapter of a book. But what I can do is give you guidelines for three basic movements and positions. If you utilize them during your workouts, this will cover probably three-quarters of your movements. I've included a video covering all three of these in the downloadable resource guide.

Basic posture

- Stand with your feet hip-width apart.
- Roll your shoulders back and down.
- Draw your ears in line with your shoulders. Chances are you may feel like you're really pulling your entire head back. Between computers and smartphones our head has become quite accustomed to tilting forward and down. Check yourself by standing against a wall and leaning the back of your heels, buttocks, shoulder blades, and back of your head on it.
- Engage your core by pulling your rib cage together (I often use the word "lacing," though this isn't actually possible) and drawing your belly button up and in. This does not mean sucking in your gut like you're trying to zip up your jeans after an indulgent season. Imagine you knew someone was going to punch you in the gut (I hope this never happens, by the way). You would contract your belly from top to bottom to protect your organs. This is essentially engaging your core.
- Keep your ears in line with your shoulders. Often we cock our head to the side when we begin to fatigue.

Plank

- Begin on your knees.
- Roll your shoulders back and engage your core (see above).
- Extend your arms straight in front of you at shoulder height.
- Lean over and place your hands on the floor directly below your shoulders.

- You should now be on all fours. Double-check your shoulders by pressing your shoulder blades down and together, and engage your core.
- Curl your toes under and straighten your legs.
- If you are new to planks, consider these options:
  - Elevate your hands to a chair or step. This takes some of the body weight off the position. Use the same tactics, and make sure your hands are still right below your shoulders.
  - Perform your plank on your knees rather than toes. If you choose this option, I recommend starting on your belly, placing your hands right by your shoulders, bending your knees so your feet are in the air, and then pushing up to extended arms. The goal is to be on the muscle above your kneecap, not on your kneecap.
- What about planks on the elbows? Yes, you can absolutely do that. The biggest form error is rounding the shoulders. Just because you are supporting yourself on your elbows doesn't give your shoulders an excuse to round forward. Keep them back and down your spine.
- Keep your ears in line with your shoulders. Look about eight-to-ten inches above your hands, and this should guide your head to where it needs to be. Do not drop your chin down or look too far up.
- Squeeze your buttocks.
- If you are planking on your toes, raise your kneecaps, which activates your quadriceps (the muscle on the front of your thigh).
- Press your heels back if you are on your toes.

Yes, I'm aware that's a heck of a lot of instructions for a plank. But considering how many bodyweight exercises are done in variations of the plank position (push-up, mountain climbers, alternating t-stands), it's worth taking the time to get it right and do it right, every time. Your body will thank you later (and hopefully you're not called out for having caved-in shoulders).

Squat

- Start with getting your basic posture correct.
- Shift your weight to your heels, bend your knees, and press your butt back like you are sitting in a chair. Make sure you can see your toes so your knees don't extend too far forward.*
- Look straight ahead or slightly up to prevent your head from dropping forward.
- Go as far down as your strength allows, working to a ninety-degree angle.
- As you straighten your legs and come back to the starting position, squeeze your glutes.
- Once your legs are fully extended, slightly tuck your hips forward to activate your hip flexors.

As I write this, I'm seeing chatter about how there is benefit to strengthening smaller muscles by actually taking your knees over your toes. There is contradicting research on its validity, and I expect more in the future. Regardless, it is proven that for general squat form to strengthen your hamstrings, glutes, and quads, you need to keep your knees behind your toes.

Cooldown

I've heard it said, "Your next workout begins at the end of your current one." The basic premise is your workout is dictated by the fueling and recovery you provide in between sweat sessions. This includes the time you invest (and it truly is an investment) in cooling down.

Just like a warm-up, a cooldown (or warm down as some coaches call it...same thing) has two components: bringing your heart rate down and elongating the muscles you just worked. If you've been working hard enough that your breathing quickens, then your heart rate is up as well. You're probably pumping that twenty to forty liters per minute we discussed earlier. The body does several things with all that blood, but basically, it's focused on cooling your heated body via sweat and moving blood to the areas that need it most like your muscles.

I often refer to the cooldown period as putting your body back together. All those adjustments it makes to get the workout done need to get back to the normal physiological state. We also need to prepare her for whatever is next on our to-do list.

How do you cool down? Depending on your goals and how you're feeling, you can try different approaches:

- *Slow down.* If you've been on a fast walk or run, take the last few minutes to decrease your pace. Then, ideally add in at least one of the next two suggestions.

- *Mobility.* We will talk more about mobility later, and I've provided the five-minute mobility cooldown I often do in the downloadable resource guide. The great thing about doing mobility at the end is it kills two birds with one stone and also offers you the benefits of joint stability, increased range of motion, and moving your body differently than you just moved it during the workout.

- *Stretch.* Now is also the time to utilize static stretching, or stretches you hold for thirty seconds or more. Dynamic stretching is also appropriate. Focus on the muscles you used the most that day or those that need some extra attention.

- *Self-myofascial release.* Also known as foam rolling, this is appropriate as a cooldown as well as a warm-up.

Now having said all this, I admit that I'm not great at taking the time to sufficiently cool down. I never claimed to be perfect. If I'm against the clock, I tend to push the workout until the last possible minute and stretch for just a couple. I pay for this in one way or the other. Don't be like me. Plan in at least five minutes of cooling down. It's also a great way of saying thank you to your body for moving it the way you asked it to. Check in with how everything feels. Respond to that. And by the way, if you're in a group fitness class and you need to hold a stretch longer than the instructor is calling for, by all means, do it.

I totally get that finding a workout online can provide inspiration and creativity. I do this too. And I understand you're motivated to jump in and do the workout without thinking too much about the other components. But don't forget them. You can still create a short, effective workout (more on this later). The most effective workouts include time for your body to ramp up and put itself back together. When you take this time, you'll decrease your chance of injury and set yourself up for another strong workout.

The Simple Take:
Adequate warming up, form, and cooldown help prevent injury and will prime your muscles for both your current workout as well as the next one. It's worth the time! Warm up with dynamic stretches, and cool down with static ones.

Five-Minute Mobility Cooldown

Check out the video in the downloadable resource guide for form instructions on planks, squats, and general posture.

Complete these movements one after the other in succession "flow." Because it's the end of the workout, you choose how long you hold each movement. I prefer to continually move, but if you have areas that are tight or need extra attention, spend more time on those. Focus on your breath as you do them, trying to coordinate one inhale or exhale for each movement.

Begin standing.

Inhale and bring your arms up.

Exhale arms down and hinge forward with a flat back.

Walk your hands out to a plank.

Bring your right foot in between your hands while keeping your left straight back.

Raise your arms straight overhead.

Bring your hands together in a prayer position, and take your left elbow over your right knee.

Raise your arms straight overhead.

Take your arms back down to the ground.

Bring your right foot to your left. You are now in a plank position.

Repeat on the other side as follows:

Bring your left foot in between your hands while keeping your right straight back.

Raise your arms straight overhead.

Bring your hands together in a prayer position, and take your right elbow over your left knee.

Raise your arms straight overhead.

Take your arms back down to the ground.

Bring your left foot to your right. You are now in a plank position.

Drop both knees to the ground.

Take your right hand above your left hand.

Press your right hip back and away from your right hand so you create a diagonal position.

Come back to all four.

Repeat on the other side as follows:

Take your left hand above your right hand.

Press your left hip back and away from your left hand so you create a diagonal position.

Come back to all fours.

Curl your toes under, and lift your hips in the sky.

Bicycle out your legs by bending one knee and straightening the other a few times each side.

Walk your hands back to your feet.

With a flat back and straight legs, return to standing.

Repeat as many times as you can within five minutes. This one feels great, so you have my permission to go longer!

CHAPTER ELEVEN

Go all in and do it right

In 2007, my friend Stephanie gave birth to her fourth child. No longer fiercely protective of her newborns, she agreed to a "meet-and-greet" baby shower a month after his arrival. We noshed on petit fours, fruit salad, and tea sandwiches. I admit celebration showers are always difficult for me. I can talk to a wall, but small chat drains the ambivert in me.

When our group of twenty sat down in a circle to watch Stephanie open presents, I breathed a sigh of relief. I don't remember any of the gifts she received, even the one from me. What I do remember is the hostess requested individual prayers over her family and newborn. She acknowledged that not everyone may feel comfortable doing this. If that was the case, guests could just stay silent and the next person would keep the chain going.

I grew up in a traditional church with guided prayers said before meals and during service. Any deviation from that in my family was a special occasion, often prepared ahead of time. My family's faith was demonstrated as the hands and feet of Jesus through actions rather than flowery, poetic prayers. And now you're asking me to come up with a prayer? On the fly? In front of twenty people? Without notes?

The blessings began, all with sweet, tender words. One after another after another, Stephanie's friends offered prayer. Each was more spiritual, more Jesus-y, more eloquent than anything I'd ever offered to God. My head bowed, I must have appeared to be deep in communion with the others. But they didn't hear my shallow breath quicken or see my glistening palms. They didn't witness the panic inside my head. Do I say something and sound like a fool, or do I remain silent? If I don't say anything, will it look like I don't care about Stephanie?

My inner hysteria heightened as the girl next to me ended with "Amen." It was my turn.

I continued sitting with my head bowed, wishing I could disappear. I could feel heads popping up like groundhogs, thinking, "Hey, it's your turn," then going back into an awkward silence. I just couldn't do it. The pressure I put on myself had intensified to a point that I felt like a failure of a friend. The girl to my right, God bless her, finally spoke up and continued the chain. In the total group, I was the only one was not comfortable or brave enough to offer a prayer for this precious newborn and his loving family.

Why didn't I just jump in and say something...anything...to keep the chain going? Why couldn't I string together a few Jesus-phrases I'd heard? Why did I feel like such a coward?

In hindsight, I believe it's because I expected that this prayer should use all the right words and scripture. I felt my words should mimic those of the women around me who had been praying out loud all their lives. I presumed I should know just the right scripture to interlace in my prayer, proving my biblical knowledge and spiritual depth. I wanted it to be perfect. Because I couldn't present that, I sat there with my head bowed in shame.

What I failed to remember, or even recognize at the time, is some of these women had been spouting off dinner blessings since before they were able to write. Many had been involved in various church ministries. And some had simply been praying this way for most of their lives.

Occasionally, women reach out to me through the privacy of email and open their hearts. They trust me with fears and frustration surrounding exercise, food, and their body. They are hurting physically, mentally, spiritually, or some combination of all three. They are exhausted. And they don't know where to start. I think they may have the same fear I had sitting in that circle: *Whatever I do or say will not be enough. And if it's not perfect, why bother? It doesn't matter how experienced or how long it's taken someone to get to where they are. I don't feel "enough" right now.*

They fear they won't be able to move like those they follow on Instagram (which, for the record, most people can't, and that is just fine). They don't know where to begin exercising. Anything they may have done in the past just doesn't seem feasible anymore. Or what they may be able to do doesn't seem to measure up to what everyone else is doing.

It's like sitting around that circle. But instead of offering praises and thanking Jesus, we listen to people talk about AMRAP, EMOM, WODs, GF, keto, and paleo. We don't feel like we can participate because we don't understand the language. Never mind the circle may consist of women who have been exercising for years or those who are in a health- or fitness-related industry. They may be nutrition geeks who love learning the science of fueling their bodies well. Health may even be a hobby, demonstrated by trying all sorts of workouts and playing around with different creations in the kitchen.

But when you're sitting in that circle and you can't offer anything, it feels like a failure without even starting. Looking back, I wish I'd offered a simple prayer for my dear friend: "Lord, thank you for Stephanie, her new baby, and their family. Help them to grow him in your love. Amen." Unfortunately, my courage wasn't there.

Since that time, I slowly started praying the words in my heart out loud. It began at the dinner table with my family. My boys were too young to recognize if what I said made sense, and my husband never showed it if he thought the prayer was awful. (Which, to be fair, no prayer is awful if it's from the heart. Some are just more fluent than others.)

My verbal prayer life grew as I led a Bible study. I established right off the bat I was uncomfortable praying out loud but would do it anyway. I stumbled and mangled my words, but I pressed on. Sixteen years later, I still don't feel eloquent or confident, but I say what's in my heart. The more I pray out loud, the more comfortable I am with it (not unlike trying a new type of movement).

Perhaps it's time we stop comparing ourselves to the seasoned health-focused people in our circle. Unless you're a gold-medal Olympic athlete, someone will always be faster, stronger, or more athletic than you. So be it.

If your health feels like me in the prayer circle, here are some strategies to consider as you figure out a realistic and sustainable program.

Start where you are

My friend Barbara and I decided to train for a half marathon together while living over five hundred miles apart. I'd been running for several years and thought it would be fun to experience. Barbara, on the other hand, regularly walked but didn't run. We each followed a training plan tailored to our skill level and checked in several times a week over text or voice memos.

What made the experience successful was each of us recognizing where our starting point was. Her plan slowly increased running distance and frequency, while mine built off of the running I already did. We each started at the right place for our fitness level. By the time race day came, we both finished with a feeling of success. I finished first, then looped back to complete the last few miles with her. We both met our goals because we respected our own starting point. That day ranks as one of my favorite all-time memories. We crossed the finish line holding hands and grinning ear to ear.

"Start where you are" is somewhat overused, but it's worth repeating. We can fall into the comparison trap if we start looking at someone else's starting point.

Begin with the easiest, then add more

When I decided I was ready to take the next step as a fitness professional and graduate from group fitness instructor to personal trainer, I did a lot of research on various programs. I settled on the National Academy of Sports Medicine (NASM). The biggest draw was the program's Optimum Performance Training (OPT) Model.

The OPT Model represents stair steps, first focusing on stabilization, then strength, then power. Guess what's easiest to start with? Stabilizing exercises. They're the foundation of all we do. I appreciated the mentality of scaling up movement for my clients and not having them immediately do exercises their bodies aren't ready for.

We take movements at one level and progress as we get stronger. For example:

- Planks with hands elevated on a chair, then knees with hands on a chair, then toes.
- Push-ups on your knees, then one foot and one knee, then two feet.
- Front- and side-laying leg lifts first, then squats.

We will get into more details on specific movements later in the next chapter.

You can use this stepwise approach with nutrition as well:

- What's the easiest evil-stepsister food to reduce (yes, the ones we talked about in "Carbs Are the Enemy")? Do that. Maybe it's cutting back to one soda a day. Then remove it completely.
- What's the easiest thing to add? Maybe it's an extra vegetable in your smoothie (try spinach or riced cauliflower). Then cut some cucumbers or buy a bag of baby carrots to grab when you need something crunchy.
- What's one plant-made food you can swap for a man-made food? Instead of those cheese-flavored crackers, try a mozzarella stick or roasted and salted chickpeas instead.

You get the point. Sometimes the most important thing is feeling successful with the easiest thing, which will, in turn, allow you to do harder things.

Embrace the uncertainty

Several years ago, a friend of mine attended my fitness class. One of the movements we did was squat jumps, and as with all my movements and classes, I showed variations. My friend chose the variation in which she elevated her heels but kept her toes on the ground. Later she confessed, "I just don't trust my body to do what it needs to do to land properly." She wasn't used to taking her body off the floor and felt uncertain about what would happen if she did. Just to be clear: You will feel weird and awkward as your body moves differently. This is normal and to be expected. What is not normal is pain and hurt, which we will discuss in "No Pain, No Gain."

When you move your body in familiar ways, it becomes efficient. The technical term for this is SAID: Specific Adaptation to Imposed Demands. Basically, your body adapts to what you're asking it to do and becomes very efficient.

When we ask our body to do something new, it's going to feel weird because it hasn't yet gained that efficiency. Our kinetic system (the chain of muscles and bones from our head to our feet) has not moved in that way before, and many new movements have to be put together to perform the new action. The bonus to inefficiency is your body becomes stronger and requires more energy as it is moved differently (in other words, you burn more calories). But just like those awkward prayers said in the privacy of my kitchen, everything starts to come together more easily. We build confidence after each uncertain step, and soon we can jump squat our way through a workout.

Experiment

My husband suffers from psoriatic arthritis. When we decided to see if removing gluten would help, we approached it as an experiment. When I proposed it, I intentionally used the word "experiment," for two reasons:

1. I truly didn't know if it would help or not.

2. Asking someone to completely eliminate their go-to foods like hamburger buns, flour tortillas, and—yes—beer is overwhelming.

I participated with him so he felt he had a partner. Plus, it didn't seem fair to dig into crusty bread in front of him. It turns out the experiment showed positive results, and we now mostly avoid gluten. My body responded with decreased inflammation, and my nagging hip injury cleared up. Of course, there are days we enjoy hamburgers and beer, but we also know we may have consequences from that.

Experimenting gives us the freedom to try something. We aren't locked in. I think that's why so many fitness programs we see specify a length of time. Whole30, P90X, and 80-Day Obsession all provide participants the opportunity to try and commit to something for a while, but—more importantly—they have a finish date. Obviously, the hope is the habit continues, but it's a lot easier starting something knowing there's an end date.

I've conducted several health-related experiments. Plant-based eating did wonders for my skin but was a lot of work, and I felt like I was on the toilet more often than not. That anti-inflammatory diet lasted until my overwhelmed breakdown. Some have lasted: gluten- and dairy-free eating gave me enough benefits that I stick by it as much as possible without being fussy. Most days I delay my first meal until 11:00 a.m., though it took me about two months to get used to intermittent fasting.

One year I experimented by trying one new-to-me fitness class per month. I danced on Kangoo boots (Google them for a smile), pounded to the beat with drumsticks, laughed at my inadequacy in a high-intensity Pilates class, and more. Knowing I was committing to one class enabled me the freedom of trying without feeling like a failure if or when I didn't return.

It's worth giving a new way of eating or movement time to sink in. When my kids were little, I read it takes twelve exposures to a new food (especially if it's a vegetable) for them to embrace it. Twelve may be overkill with a particular class, but I recommend giving it at least three times. In my early twenties, I closed the door on yoga because I was so confused and uncomfortable the first time I tried it. I also didn't feel I got a "real workout" in because I wasn't sweaty and breathing hard. (If only I'd known how helpful it was.) Fast forward a few years, and when I tried it again (this time with more consistency), it stuck.

Consider creating a plan to experiment with your food or movement. Yes, it's helpful to plan when that will be and what that will look like. But just as important is allowing yourself the flexibility to try something and assess from there.

Habit stack

Habit stacking, or combining habits with another habit you are currently executing, was first introduced by BJ Fogg and popularized by James Clear's *Atomic Habits.* The concept is to take something you already do and attach a habit to it. The formula is "after/before [current habit], I will [new habit]."

For example: After lunch, I will meditate. Before dinner, I will make sure I've consumed all my water throughout the day (bonus: fewer bathroom trips at night!).

(Notice this formula does not say new habits. Habit = singular. Find one change and figure out how to implement that into your current routine. Then add another one.)

My habits change with the seasons. As a mom of two teen boys, I've viewed the beginning of the school year as the most impactful time I can establish new habits. Coming off the summer months, when flexibility and spontaneity are the names of the game, I find myself craving structure and routine. I also cherish the routines I keep, like my coffee and Jesus time. No matter the time of year, this time centers me and makes me a better wife and mother. Without it, I just feel off.

I'd like to say my prayer time is intentional and fervent each day. Sometimes it is. Sometimes, though, it consists of reading a chapter in the Bible or whatever study I'm in, then losing my thoughts in the presence of Jesus. Not engaging in deep conversation with Him, but just following some kind of rabbit trail of what's on my heart or agenda for the day. I imagine He patiently waits for me, wishing I would land the plane. I'm not always great at keeping the focus, and I lose track of time. This is where it gets tricky. I cherish my morning quiet time, but sometimes it extends too long, and then I'm slivering off other parts of my calendar.

Enter that season's habit formula. I found if I worked out *before* my Jesus time, I stayed on track. My exercise had firmer time boundaries. After all, as much as I love to move my body, I also try to get in and out of the gym (or walk, run, etc.) as efficiently as possible. Scheduling forty-five minutes to exercise, *then* sitting down with coffee, Jesus, and often a sweat towel keeps me on track.

Hire a coach

Some people thrive on structure. If you feel the need to develop some sort of a plan, consider hiring a coach or asking a friend who knows what she's doing. You will not be surprised to hear me say I recommend a personal trainer, who can give you the personal attention you deserve and may need. If she's worth the weight of her certificate, she should take your individual needs and expectations into consideration. I enjoy working with clients who have issues we need to work around. Finding creative ways to strengthen the quads and hamstrings of a client who has arthritis gives me a strange pleasure. The other nice thing about a personal trainer? You don't have to do any thinking. You show up and do what she tells you to do. You don't have to plan. She does it all.

One option growing in popularity is small-group private training. Some call this "share the trainer." If you buddy up with two or three friends, you can probably find a trainer who is willing to work with your group. You should pay a discounted rate from the personal training session, and the trainer will earn more. It's a win-win.

I'd be remiss not to mention choosing a *Certified* Personal Trainer, one who has gone through a full program and been tested for her certification. Experience speaks volumes, but so does immersing oneself in understanding the musculature system and how it works together. New research and studies are constantly evolving. We fitness professionals must receive continuing education credits to stay certified, so you'll be ensured yours is abreast of the latest discoveries. A trainer can spot nuances in the way your body moves and strengthen those areas. She can also make sure your form is correct so you don't risk injuring yourself. Yes, you can get this in a group fitness setting, but at a much lower level. It's difficult to tweak twenty clients during coaching a class.

Fitness comes second nature to me. Nutrition is my Achilles' heel. Hiring a nutrition coach was one of the most impactful decisions I've made concerning my eating. You'll hear more of this story later. Yes, there was a plan to start, but I didn't have to come up with it. She provided guidance and grace in equal amounts. When our official time was over, I acquired sustainable tools I could use myself. I hired her before becoming certified myself, but I can honestly say having someone to encourage me and keep me accountable was invaluable.

There's an element of ego-swallowing that comes with hiring someone or asking for help. As a fitness professional, I feel like I should know it all. I don't. I'm also human and need support. Yes, I lean on Jesus. I also lean on people He put in my life.

If a personal trainer isn't in the cards and you're comfortable with your form, consider finding a friend who has some experience under her belt. You'd be surprised how willing people are to share their knowledge with you.

Sitting in that prayer circle so many years ago, I never imagined myself leading women through prayer (at speaking events, no less). Are those prayers eloquent and powerful? Of course not. But I have the confidence to speak my heart now. What felt insurmountable before is now comfortable. The same is true as you begin new healthy habits. They may feel impossible, but taking small steps will make you more comfortable and confident in your efforts.

If you're not used to moving or fueling your body with God's foods, you're not alone. It's overwhelming. Try just one of these tactics. The only expectation you need to meet is that of finding something that works for you. Then, just like those simple prayers that are now longer and spoken more easily, you can find the best way to take care of your body.

The Simple Take:
You don't need to have a solid plan before beginning a health journey. Experiment with different tactics and strategies until you find what works for you.

CHAPTER TWELVE

Working out is too complicated

Sipping a Moscow Mule, I found myself discussing exercise with my husband's coworker. Yes, friends, this is the beginning of great health conversations: at a bar. Whilst consuming vodka, ginger beer, and a splash of lime. The irony. Yet there we sat, while my husband was deep in conversation with someone else. It was January, and this coworker was saying how hard it had been to get back into "health mode" this year. Not the least of his challenges were his four children under the age of eight and the time demands of being a father, husband, and primary income earner.

"I need to talk to your husband about working out," he stated. "He seems to know a lot about it and does a good job of exercising. Quite honestly, I go into the gym or find myself staring at the weights in my garage, and I don't know where to begin. I just don't know how to work out. It's too complicated. Maybe he can help me."

I wasn't quite sure how to respond to that. Yes, my husband does have a solid level of knowledge around the fundamentals of exercise. And I understand this coworker would probably prefer the advice of another dude. After all, my focus is on women around my age. But I couldn't help but feel somewhat insulted.

"You know I'm a personal trainer, right?" I replied with a gentle smile.

He did not know this. I tried not to be hurt. These men have worked together for *ten years,* and it never came out that I'm a fitness professional? Perhaps I will give my loving husband the benefit of the doubt and trust he's mentioned it, but the coworker didn't remember amidst all his other responsibilities.

He spoke the truth of so many, though. Here's a little-known secret: many people, regardless of their fitness level, do not feel they know how to work out. They know how to show up at the gym. They know how to watch Instagram or YouTube videos. They may even know how to amp up their intensity in a group fitness class. But if they were to walk onto the floor of a gym, they might look around, see all of the various equipment and torture machines, get overwhelmed, and leave. Or, more likely, they might just find themselves on a treadmill or elliptical machine just to get some moving in. (Which there is no shame in, but it doesn't help you achieve a well-rounded workout.)

I understand. It seems like the gym environment has its own language. AMRAP, WOD, supersets, lions and tigers and bears, oh my! It's confusing. I confess: I contribute to this madness. Fitness geeks such as myself relish learning new ways to move our bodies. Exercise science is my passion. Because it is also my job, I find it only responsible to keep abreast of all of the latest techniques, research, and quirky language.

The problem is we can easily complicate matters for people who just want to take care of themselves.

You can find a million different ways to move your body. Some require more flexibility than others; some require more strength. Some are creative; others are simple. Some are just flat-out crazy impressive. One of these days, I'm hoping to be able to properly replicate some of the impressive shots from the Athleta fitness clothing magazines. It's unlikely, though.

Rather than breaking this rule for you, I want to give you the tools and resources to break it yourself. No more staring at weights and bands, not knowing what to do with them. We are done brushing off strength day because we're unclear what to do. (Worried about bulking up? Tune into the next chapter).

Take comfort in knowing there is no one right or wrong way to work out. Yes, I do want your form to be right, as we covered earlier. But the main workout part where you get 'er done? It really doesn't have to be complicated.

The right way is the one you'll do consistently. But to be consistent, you need to show up with enough confidence to execute it. Let's go back to the problem at hand. *How exactly does one work out when they don't know where to begin?* If that is how you are feeling, I'm here to help. I'm also going to assume you are not trying to enter a fitness competition or qualify for the Olympics. You just want to take care of your body. We don't need to get too technical. We just need to strengthen our muscles, get our heart beating faster, and be able to move our joints in all the directions they were meant to move. (I can't wait for you to try the mobility set provided in Chapter 18: "There's One Right Way to Exercise.")

I'm also going to assume you don't have a fully stocked gym at your house. You are probably trying to sandwich fitness in between your morning alarm clock and coffee or between work and dinner. We aren't going to get too crazy here. We are just going to go over the basics.

Create space

First, create space. All you need is about eight feet by eight feet. Here are some ideas to create this space if it's not staring you in the face:

- Move the coffee table.
- Head to the garage (but maybe not for high-impact workouts).
- Use your college-aged children's room (they'll never know).
- Head to your back porch.
- Find a grassy spot outside.

Move your body in all directions

Next, recognize your body is meant to move in all directions. Up and down, forward and backward, side to side, and diagonally. We will cover this more later in the book. This is important for two reasons:

1. Moving in many directions helps prevent overuse and injury.

2. Embracing that your body can move in practically any direction frees you to try movements without fear of being "wrong."

Understand the basic modalities

Walking onto a gym floor can be ridiculously overwhelming. Some of the equipment and machines have perfectly good uses but also look a little bit like torture machines. Let's cover some of the more recognizable ones, bearing in mind that terms may vary from trainer to trainer:

- *Resistance loops.* These are typically circular stretchy bands that are ten to twelve inches in circumference. They are about two inches thick and basically look like a huge rubber band. If you've ever been to physical therapy you may have used these, though they can also be used in your general workouts. I use resistance loops with my teen clients as they are at a low price point (around $8–$10) for a set of five different resistances.

- *Resistance bands.* These are longer stretchy bands often about three feet long with handles. Resistance bands are another favorite of mine as you can get a set of five for about $35 and create your own resistance. My favorite set is one that has fabric covering over the plastic bands. It has interchangeable handles, which is helpful in customizing resistance, as well as a door anchor to customize where you want the anchor point. I can also interlace two bands on one handle and increase the challenge.

- *Kettlebells.* Kettlebells have been around since 1885 and for good reason. They offer a variety of uses. Because the weight is offset between the handle and the "bell," they challenge your muscles differently. Picture a circular weight with a handle. When you hold a kettlebell, it may rock back and forth. This inconsistent weight distribution helps challenge your core and smaller stabilizing muscles.

- *Dumbbells.* More than likely you envision dumbbells when you hear the phrase "strength training." These have equal weight on either end of a shorter straight bar. One hand typically holds one dumbbell.

- *Barbells.* These steel bars are longer, between three and four feet. They are designed to stack weight plates on either end and used for movements for larger and stronger muscle groups. You may use these for a chest press or squats.

- *Machines.* Machines are intended to isolate specific muscles. If you look at any machine in your local gym, it will often include a graphic that highlights the muscle(s) the machine helps you work on. Machines can be less intimidating than they look because they often include specific how-to instructions and visuals.

- *Bodyweight.* Yes, you can absolutely get an effective and challenging workout by using your body. I can take my 146 pounds and do all kinds of exercises to strengthen my muscles.

Feel free to try other ones not listed, but more than likely, the list above will fit your needs.

What do we do with the different modalities?

If you're interested in trying the above equipment but confused about where to start or how much weight or resistance to use, I highly recommend a session or two with a Certified Personal Trainer who can walk you through everything. Some gyms offer this as a complimentary service when you join.

Types of movement

Movement patterns, in which we mimic actual movements, utilize several muscles at once (great for calorie-burning as well if that's a goal of yours). They also reduce the tendency to overdevelop muscles, causing imbalance or injury (which should be a goal of yours).

Let's talk about some of the foundational knowledge and then how you can create workouts even if you don't know how to work out.

There are six basic types of movement patterns:

1. Push
2. Pull
3. Squat
4. Hinge
5. Lunge/single leg
6. Rotational

Push

Pushing involves moving your hands away from you to the front or overhead. Visualize a push-up. Another is an overhead press. In this movement, you stand with your feet together or on one foot for bonus balance work. Bend your elbows into a ninety-degree angle, and place them at shoulder height with your palms facing out. To keep your shoulders safe, it's recommended your elbows are in front of your face.[1] With dumbbells in your hands, press up over your head and back down, returning to your original position. Even though the weight is going up, you are still pushing it away from your body.

Pull

Pulling, by contrast, involves moving your hands toward your body from the front or an overhead position. Pull-ups are an obvious example of this. Your hands are overhead grasping a bar and you pull them toward your body, which lifts your body toward the bar. I would love to tell you how to do this, but this is not something I have accomplished. Pull-ups are awful and horrid, and I stand in awe and wonder of those who can complete more than a handful of reps. If you are like me and can't do more than one or two pull-ups (if that), you can utilize resistance bands to simulate this motion. Anchor your band above your head, and pull down. You can also execute pulling motions in your lower body. If you've ever utilized prone leg curl machines to lay on your belly ("prone" position), place your ankles under a padded bar, and bring your heels toward your rear, this, too, is a pulling motion.

Squat

Squatting means your feet are in contact with the ground and your hips flex while they draw down closer to your feet. Yes, you can do squats on a squat machine, but I prefer the machine-free version of standing on the ground. There are many progressions of a squat, but an effective one is the basic squat. Standing with your feet hip-width apart, shoulders rolled back and core engaged, sit your rear back like you are sitting in a chair. Watch your knees to make sure they do not go over your toes. You want your butt to go back, but you don't want your knees to lean forward beyond your toes, especially if you are adding resistance. As you come up, squeeze your glutes and then slightly press your hips forward at the top. Squat complete. Repeat, and add weight by using dumbbells or resistance bands as your legs strengthen.

Hinge

Hinging occurs mostly in your hips. Just like a door hinge has one moving part (the door) and a stabilizing unity (the frame), your upper body can hinge downward while your legs stay straight. If you've ever bent down to stretch your legs in a standing position, this is a hinge. Kettlebell swings are also hinging movements.

Lunge/single leg

Lunge and single-leg movements have to do with one foot leaving the ground while the other leg is doing the work. Begin with your feet together and then take a wide step backward. Drop your hips until your front leg is at a ninety-degree angle, or go as far as is comfortable for you. Bring your back leg up to your front then do the same thing on the other side.

Rotational

Rotational movements are a current favorite of mine. They involve rotating either your thoracic spine, which is your middle back, or your pelvis. A simple spinal twist, in which you stand with your feet hip-width apart and simply rotate your shoulders back and forth to either side, is a great way to warm up. Rotational movements are important to include in your movement as they can help strengthen your core and prevent injury.

Now you know the six basic movements, but what do you do with them? Find a few movements in each category, and rotate through them. Ideally, follow a pattern that uses opposite movements. Push, then pull. Or squat, then rotate. Giving opposite muscles equal playing time prevents you from looking like Popeye, with his bulky forearms and stick upper arms (pre-spinach power, of course). More importantly, it prevents overtraining particular muscles and/ or creating a muscle imbalance.

A quick lesson on muscle imbalance: Imagine taking two Jenga blocks and leaning them upright against each other to create an upside-down "V." This represents your muscles providing equal resistance and pressure, or muscle balance. If we were to place more weight on one piece, the "V" would lean to the side. It would pull anything connected to it, causing spasms, strains, or other issues. In other words: muscle imbalance is not good.

If executing the six types of movements has your head spinning, consider a different approach. Compartmentalize your exercises into one of four categories: upper body, lower body, core, and cardio.

If you're not sure which category exercises fall under, or even what to do, these are all available on the free resource guide. There, you may download a cheat sheet of both the types of movements (push/

pull/squat/hinge/lunge/rotational) and areas of the body (upper, lower, cardio, core).

How many reps should you do? Good question. I recommend starting with eight to ten repetitions of any movement. If you fly through and finish the tenth rep without any difficulty, it's time to add more reps or increase your weight by 10 percent.

Finally, just like with carbohydrates, know you can have too much of a good thing. Allow your muscles forty-eight hours in between strength sessions to allow for repair and recovery. Factor in rest days. And make sure you tune into the later chapter "No Rest for the Weary."

Remember: The most effective workout is one you will do consistently and that leaves you feeling equal parts energized, fatigued, and accomplished. These are good starting points, but ultimately, you have control over how you move. Consider these suggestions to get you started on how to work out. In the meantime, I'll have this on hand for next time I'm sipping a Moscow Mule and hear, "I don't know how to work out."

The Simple Take:
You don't need to have a full understanding of all modalities, machines, and movements. Use some of the basic ones provided here, and when in doubt,
just move your body.

Functional Movement Workout

Following are movements that fall in the functional movement category. This is not a comprehensive list! I tried to choose exercises that are adequately executed through your own body weight or through resistance bands. If you have other forms of resistance (e.g., dumbbells), then by all means, use those.

Proper form is demonstrated through the link in the free downloadable resource guide.

Push
1. Lying band chest press
2. Push-ups
3. Band flye
4. Standing band chest press

Pull
1. Bent-over row
2. Band pull down
3. Reverse flye
4. Prone band lateral extension pulls

Squat
1. Squat
2. Plie squat
3. Goblet squat
4. Sumo squat

Hinge
1. Deadlifts
2. Single-leg deadlifts
3. Good mornings
4. Kettlebell swings

Lunge/Single Leg
1. Single-leg sit to stand
2. Single-leg squat w/reach
3. Lateral lunge

Rotational
1. Diagonal lunge
2. High-to-low band chop*
3. Low-to-high band chop*
4. Bicycles

*When you "chop," you bring your straight arms diagonally from one side to the other. High to low means you start high on one side and bring it down to the other. Low to high is the opposite. Both of these are demonstrated in the free resource guide.

To plan a workout, choose one of these combinations:

- Push/Pull;
- Squat/Hinge
- Lunge or Single Leg/Rotational

Perform alternating numbers in each combination (1, 1, 2, 2, 3, 3, etc.). For example, in a push/pull workout, do lying band chest press, bent-over row, push-ups, band pull down, etc. Do each movement 8 times, working your way up to 20 reps, before moving on to the next.

For **more** intensity focus on only one combination, and repeat the round for a total of 2–5 times. For **less** intensity, go through all three combinations.

Area Focus: Bodyweight Workout

Upper	Lower	Core	Cardio
1. Push-ups	1. Squats	1. Plank	1. Plank jacks
2. Tricep dips	2. Reverse lunges	2. Floor prone cobra	2. Squat jumps
3. Bear crawl	3. Diagonal lunges	3. Alternating t-stand	3. High knees

To construct a workout, try one of the following:

First, warm up at least 5 minutes. See the resource guide for a full-body warm-up tutorial.

- Perform all 1s, 2s, then 3s. Start with :25 seconds, working up to :60 seconds.
  or
- Perform each category in order. All upper, all lower, all core, all cardio. Start with :25 seconds and break as needed, working up to :60 seconds.

CHAPTER THIRTEEN

I don't want to bulk up

Over the years, I've had numerous women approach me after class. "I love your arms," they'll say. "I really want to strengthen mine and be able to wear sleeveless tops. But I don't want to get too strong. I don't want to bulk up.

Because my self-image journey is ever-present, my head creates an internal dialogue: *Does she want arms like mine? Or is she saying they're too bulky? Is she saying I'm too bulky overall? Like, Amy, I want your arms but not your bulk? You're too strong?*

I never said this dialogue was helpful. It just exists. Still, most days I can admit I have great arms. I had Michelle Obama arms before Michelle Obama arms were a thing. Oh goodness, I did not just one-up the former First Lady. This is the woman who defied tradition and posed sleeveless (*Gasp!*) in her official First Lady photo. Her gorgeous inauguration dress foreshadowed this with a white, one-shouldered display. Through her eight years in the White House, her arms became a full-on *thing*, and God bless her she wasn't afraid to show them.

Her book *Becoming* discussed her journey to begin exercising. Her reasoning? The same as most clients I work with: she just wanted to take care of herself. And in the process, she created gorgeous arms.

In the sixteen years I've been a fitness leader, women (thankfully) have begun to embrace strength. #StrongWomen currently holds over fifteen million tags on Instagram. Social media influencers flaunt their strength with impressive moves or by flexing their back, quad, and yes, bicep muscles. Still, we seem to meet this with mixed emotions. We want that strength. We want the ability to demonstrate individual muscles when flexed. But there's a resistance to being "bulky." We want to be strong but not "too" strong.

While the geeky trainer in me wants to immediately throw out a bunch of facts and science as to why it's difficult to bulk up, I think it's important to dig into the statement "I don't want to bulk up."

What does "bulky" mean to you?

If you're looking for a specific answer to that, you're going to be disappointed. For some, "bulky" may reference large deltoids (shoulders) protruding from a sleeveless shirt. For others, the term may mean filling out her jeans with curvy thighs or having biceps visible under a long-sleeve shirt.

The truth is one woman's "bulk" is another woman's "defined muscle." What may be "too much" for you isn't enough for another. My hope is we can be comfortable in the optimal size for our body when we fuel it well and move it properly. Sometimes I'm there myself; sometimes I have to take those negative thoughts captive and reframe them with positive thoughts about my body.

Perhaps "bulky" is a fear of not having a body that's enough. Thin enough, lean enough, attractive enough. In the same breath, I'd like to offer two conflicting responses: I get it, and enough of this madness. I've fought the same battle in my mind. I still do sometimes. The only way I beat the madness is by embracing the uniquely created body God gave me and reminding myself I'm able to live out those callings we talked about in Chapter 2.

Why do you think you'll bulk up?

At some point in the early nineties, I remember the Queen of Pop, Madonna, taking the stage at an awards show. She stepped onstage to deliver or accept an award. However, no one talked about the award, only her shoulders and biceps. They appeared huge. My high school friends and I agreed: she was too bulky. I know, I just told you not to use that word. But this was thirty years ago, and the mindset of "be thin, lean, and attractive" consumed me.

Somehow my mind decided I would look bulky if I strength trained. Maybe you've experienced a similar connection. I'll share the difference between strength training and growing your muscles in a minute. But first, let me tell you why strength training is important.

Why do I want you strength training anyway?

I place a strong focus on strength training (also called resistance training) with the women I train, most of whom are over forty. I care less about how big their biceps are and focus more on functional muscles. As we age, it's important to strengthen the muscles we use on a daily basis so we can do the things we love to do. Resistance training for women offers many benefits:

- It increases resting metabolic rate (otherwise known as metabolism). One study showed an estimated 5 percent increase after nine months.[1]
- It increases bone density in postmenopausal women.[2]
- It helps to manage high blood pressure. One study showed that an eight-week resistance training program performed three times a week positively reduces peripheral blood pressure (taken with an arm cuff) and enhances the degree in which blood vessels fully open.[3] The clients in this program performed alternating upper-body and lower-body exercises in a circuit (also known as peripheral heart action). By the way, it's worth noting that for the safety of the prehypertensive and hypertensive client, do not resistance train to failure. In other words, don't bench-press until you can't get the weights up anymore.
- It decreases the average blood-sugar levels in diabetic women and men.[4] Additionally, increasing muscle mass can help glycogen (energy) be stored in the muscles of type 2 diabetics.[5] If you or a loved one has type 2 diabetes and has been told to

control your blood sugar, increasing your muscles can help this.

- It increases carbohydrate/glycogen metabolism from the type II muscle fibers (type II is what your body develops with strength training). You know that occasional dessert we don't have to work off? Your muscles will help do that for you if you've been strength training.

- It increases levels of human growth hormones, which can help metabolize free fatty acids. Why do we care about those? They can help the skin appear younger. Yes, please. I need all the help I can get in this area.

You may have already heard some of these benefits. Perhaps you already incorporate strength training into your week. (If so, good for you!) But maybe, somewhere deep down, you...I...want to avoid the stigma of being bulky. If that's the case, please consider the following.

1. There's a difference between strength training and hypertrophy

You can get stronger without creating hypertrophy (increasing your muscle size) and vice versa. Your skeletal muscles (those on the main part of your body, as opposed to your heart/cardiac muscle) respond differently based on the load and speed they are being asked to perform. Your goals will dictate your training program.

Those training for *hypertrophy* utilize a higher-volume strategy of greater loads (weight) and fewer reps. For example, if I were trying to increase my pectoral (chest) size, I might bench-press thirty-pound dumbbells between six and eight times to reach fatigue. Heavy load, few reps.

In contrast, *training for muscular strength endurance* achieves less hypertrophy but still results in increased strength. It also increases lean body mass and enhances joint stabilization. In the same chest-press example, I might grab the twenty-pound weights and perform eight to twelve reps. Lower weight, more reps. This is applicable in many physical therapies as well. My bum shoulder requires a low-load, high-rep workout to stabilize the muscles. It should be noted you will still see some muscle definition with strength training, particularly if you are just starting. But to get those extra-big muscles, you'll need to shift your approach to higher load and fewer reps rather than moderate load and more reps.

If you have specific goals, particularly hypertrophy, I recommend finding a Certified Personal Trainer who can partner with you. But first, review the section on Certified Personal Trainers in the chapter "Go All In and Do It Right" to make sure you find the right one. If he's wearing a "*Pass the Bucket*" tank, it's best you pass.

Otherwise, strength train your heart out without fear of getting "bulky." Grab some weights that are appropriate for you to perform eight to twelve reps, where you fatigue by the end. If you blow through fifteen reps, it's time to increase your weight by about 10 percent. Remember: If you struggle with high blood pressure, stop before you get to the point of failure so you don't strain at the end.

2. Getting "bulky" takes enormous discipline outside of the gym

We all have biceps. If you have two legs, or even just one, you have four muscles on the front of each leg that make up your quadriceps. And yes, you have a six-pack (even if you can't see it), which is actually eight when considering the full *rectus abdominous*. We all have the same muscles. However, no matter how much focus I put into strength and/or hypertrophy, I will have a hard time showing off those muscles if I haven't exhibited the same discipline in the kitchen as in the gym.

The quality and quantity of the food we eat can have an enormous impact on our physique. This is not news to anyone. But consider what it means to prominently display our muscles. First, we must find ourselves regularly lifting heavy weight.

With the help of Google, I reviewed some images of Madonna during this period of time. What I see now are defined muscles. I also see an extremely lean body. If she felt great in her body, then more power to her. And knowing Madonna, she did. She also may have had additional resources available to pop queens like dietitians and personal chefs to menu plan and prep. They may have diligently created high-protein, calorie-restrictive meals and most certainly didn't buy cookies "for the kids" as I do. Most importantly, she probably didn't allow herself any indulgence or leeway in her nutrition. This is speculation, of course. But I can tell you this: I have no desire or the time to put in that kind of discipline to be that lean.

If we want each muscle to pop, we have to ensure there is not too much adipose tissue between said muscles and our skin. In essence, our body fat needs to remain low. While strength training absolutely contributes to our metabolism by increasing the basal metabolic rate, or the rate at which we burn calories while resting, it is not the only contributing factor to adipose. We also must decrease our energy intake (obtained by food) to lose some of that tissue. Of course, we still need enough energy to perform said strength training and go about our everyday lives.

That's a lot of work, by the way.

Gaining strength takes discipline. The reality is that bulking up, in the sense of showing off those muscles, is no easy task. I have to increase my energy and particularly my protein enough to meet the needs of my muscles but at the same time reduce my intake to eliminate fat. It's possible, for sure. However it's not something that happens passively or even with just a couple of strength training sessions per week.

3. Your body predisposition will guide your muscle mass

Back to my arms. When clients compliment me, I typically respond by telling them my toned deltoids, biceps, and triceps are a combination of hard work and genetics, more heavily weighted on the latter. Then I share how my mother (whose age I won't share, but she's old enough to have a forty-six-year-old daughter) has amazing arms without doing any toning or strengthening exercises. Yes, she does take care of herself by using the elliptical machine and side-stroke swimming, but not a pound of steel is intentionally lifted. She bestowed her great arms on me, just like my face structure and height.

My children, like yours, are wonderfully made. God created each of them with intent and as unique as you and I are. They resemble each other in their smile, height, and blond hair. At twenty months apart, my younger son is referred to as his older brother's "mini-me." Their personalities are not quite as congruent, but that's what makes things fun.

They both tower over me. My five-foot-four frame now looks up to my children who are currently six-foot-five and six-foot-two. Don't tell anyone, but we are gunning for the younger one to outpace his brother on the height chart. My older son has always received the most attention about his height, and we think it'd be funny to have his little brother a sliver higher by the time it's all said and done. We are a little twisted that way.

While both consistently chart over 90 percent at the doctor's office, their weight curves show a different trajectory. My older son's height and weight curves are parallel. My younger son, however, shows a gap. His weight has never tracked as high as his height.

This discrepancy has nothing to do with their activity level or food intake. They are simply built differently. From the neck down, my younger son is the spitting image of my husband: long and lean.

The older one, on the other hand, received his father's height (and some of my father's as well) but has a lot of muscle packed into his body, just like me. His legs make my muscular thighs seem waiflike and his primary complaint is he has a hard time getting sore after leg workouts. His younger brother, on the other hand, could run his cross-country meets with a brick between his legs and not have a problem. I never understood how inherent our body frames are from the moment we are born until I had more than one child. I saw this from the first few diapers I changed. Even their teeny-tiny bottoms fit their newborn-sized diapers differently.

Sixteen years later, I see this in their physiques. While both see results from their gym work, they are exhibited differently. The older one seems to show his strength more easily. His predisposed musculature puffs up within a few weeks. Long and lean's body is sneaky. His frame hides his muscles until one day he takes his shirt off to swim or cool down and bam, there's a gun show going on.

The last few summers, I've been teaching a teen fitness class. It's something I fell into that God knew I needed. These young women want to move and take care of themselves. While I appreciate that they are scouring YouTube and Instagram for ideas and workouts, the trainer and educator in me wants to make sure they are executing the movements properly so they don't get hurt.

They arrived at various fitness levels with different foundations. One of my girls was the poster child for using great form. Quiet and respectful, she responded to my comments with "Yes ma'am." In particular, she executed push-ups perfectly on her knees. I could tell she was getting stronger, but she didn't quite have the confidence to progress.

One day I bent down and gently asked, "Can you try something for me? Take those push-ups out to your toes. Let's just see what happens." Sure enough, she completed ten push-ups...on her toes...with precision. I tried to balance my enthusiasm with her quiet demeanor. I failed. Nor could she contain her wide smile. She was proud of herself. She captured something she didn't know she would do and took a big step in increasing her confidence that day.

When your trainer tells you to grab the twenty-pound dumbbells rather than the fifteens you've been using, try it. Consider it even if you are your own trainer. See what happens. You may find yourself pleasantly surprised at what you can handle. Your trainer sees strength in you. She wants you to feel it as well. Don't let your fear of bulk get in the way.

The Simple Take:
Strength training offers internal and external benefits,
and more than likely will not leave you looking "bulky."
Allow yourself to see what happens when you
lift heavy things.

30-Minute Full-Body Strength Workout

If I've convinced you to strength train but you're not sure where to begin, try this full-body thirty-minute workout. Use this page to guide your workout, or join me in the video provided in the downloadable resource guide.

Warm-Up

30 seconds each, two rounds:

- Loop walks (or duck walks if you don't have resistance loops)
- Twists
- Squats
- Bear crawls
- Push-ups on knees

Set

Perform each movement 40 seconds, then take a 20-second break. Begin with two rounds, making your way up to four complete rounds. If 40 seconds is too long, begin with 25 seconds of work with a 20-second break. Increase your weight with each round.

- Squat with overhead press (elbows in)
- Renegade row
- Alternating reverse lunges with lateral extension (thumbs-up)
- Scissors
- Push-up walks
- Headbangers with legs in tabletop
- Deadlift to hammer curl

Cooldown

30 seconds each:

- Chest opener
- Pigeon on right side
- Pigeon on left side
- Supine spinal twist, right
- Supine spinal twist, left
- Ankle and wrist rolls
- Gentle rolls
- Sitting deep breaths

CHAPTER FOURTEEN

I have to get my hour of exercise in

_M_y first memory of attending a group fitness class includes a royal-blue thong leotard and black biker shorts. My seventeen-year-old self was embarking on her first "grown-up" foray into the fitness world, having graduated from the elliptical machines on the gym floor to attempting a step aerobics class. I need not tell you this was the early 90s; step aerobics was all the rage, and those horrid thong leotards accompanied it. (_What were we thinking?_) My friend and I made plans to meet each other at the 7:00 p.m. step aerobics class.

We arrived early. Looking through the classroom's glass wall, we watched the previous class stretching their hamstrings by placing one heel on the step and leaning back into the other foot. Next, they elevated onto the step and lowered their heels off, one at a time, to lengthen their calf muscles.

At 6:55 p.m., when the instructor provided the verbal cue they were done, the class clapped—For themselves? For the instructor? Thirty years later, I'm still not sure why we still do this—and began gathering their items to depart. The uber-dedicated remained on their step, ready for part two of their workout.

Over the next five minutes, the fresh crew shuffled in, staked their claim at their preferred steps, and adjusted them as necessary. Right on the dot, at 7:00 p.m., the steady thirty-two-count beat began, and we followed instructions for right step, left step, step knee, and around the world. Fifty-five-minutes later, it was our turn to clap. We walked our sweaty selves back to our car to resume life.

This fifty-five-minute rhythm was ingrained in my mind so much that if we got into the classroom a few minutes late or—heaven forbid—class ended three minutes early, I felt ripped off. Apparently, the magic fifty-five-minute number validated my efforts. Fifty-two minutes was not nearly enough. I had to hit that fifty-five minutes.

Fast-forward thirty years, and you'll rarely find me formally exercising more than forty minutes. Most of the time, it's closer to thirty. What changed? Well, for one I got older, and my body just doesn't like those long sweat sessions. Time is more valuable. But I also learned to retrain my brain along with learning the latest science supporting shorter workouts. I can achieve a solid workout in less than an hour. You can too.

As our country has become more sedentary over the last forty years, our government leaders have tried to encourage us to move. I'd be remiss not to specifically mention former First Lady Michelle Obama, who led us through the "Let's Move" White House campaign encouraging our youth to turn off the Xbox and find joy in movement. Politics aside, you can't argue that she made hula hooping and gardening look cool.

After all, we were meant to move. Think back to biblical days. Jesus and His disciples walked countless miles (in leather straps, mind you, not the orthopedic stabilizers I wear all the time). Before that, we hunted and gathered food. Sustaining life required our bodies to move. When we migrated to computers and desks, we needed a bit of a kick in the butt to get us up and moving. Fifty-five minutes of formal exercise seemed like just the right prescription. Sitting ten hours a day? No worries. Simply schedule in an hour on top of commuting, work, kids' practices, dinner prep, dinner, and heaven forbid a little time with your spouse before calling it a night. Check the hour off your box and you're good. Also exhausted.

You probably already have a full day without throwing an hour of exercise in the mix. For rule followers such as myself, there's a shame that can go along with not accomplishing it. If you're a perfectionist on top of that, you probably think, "If I can't get an hour in, then it's not worth it."

Let's ditch the one-hour mentality. And just for grins, let's throw some research into the mix so you can stand firm on your shorter workout.

Following are a few points to consider as you give yourself the freedom to not work out a full hour.

Something is better than nothing

In 2008, the US Department of Health and Human Services (HHS) realized our society was becoming more sedentary and released guidelines on how often to move. The guidelines were designed to provide information and guidance on the types and amounts of physical activity that provide substantial health benefits.

The HHS guidelines tell me that for substantial health benefits, I should do 150 to 300 minutes of moderately intense exercise per week. Alternatively, I can achieve seventy-five minutes of vigorous-intensity aerobic physical activity.[1] Broken down, this is a thirty-minute power walk five days a week. Or hit it hard for twenty-five minutes every Monday, Wednesday, and Friday (see below for more on why this shorter time is beneficial).

I like rules. While the concept of this book contradicts this, I find peace in knowing what I am supposed to do. If you tell me substantial health benefits are achieved through a formula, my instinct is to make sure I check off my minutes. The forty-five-minute classes and training sessions I coach start and end right on time (most days).

For many of us rule followers, we tend to think if we can't get in the recommended amount of time we need or expect, then we ought not proceed. No time for that hour? We tell ourselves, "Don't even bother. If you can't do it right, don't do it at all. If the day's goal is thirty-five minutes but we can only fit in twenty-eight, then it's not worth it."

This is nonsense. Twenty-eight minutes count. So do thirty, twenty, even ten.

In fact, the latest research shows even eleven minutes of exercise is beneficial. A study reported in the *British Journal of Sports Medicine* found that those who achieved eleven minutes of moderate-to-vigorous exercise were less likely to die than those who only exercised two minutes.[2] Considering the subjects had daily activities that found them sitting eight to ten hours a day, this is encouraging. Suddenly, getting in that workout on top of all our daily activities seems more doable.

It's time to lose the one-hour rule. Those fifty-five-minute classes work well in creating gym schedules. However, if they aren't conducive to your routine, then figure out what is. Remember, the intent behind those HHS physical activity guidelines is to get people up and moving. I know I can be guilty of being fairly sedentary on days I am working on several computer-based tasks. Between writing, podcast prep, podcast recording, and all of the other one-off projects, I find my butt in a chair way too often. This is not okay. Squeezing in half an hour, or even eleven minutes, helps get my body set to sit.

Your favorite HIIT workout might better serve you shortened

High-intensity interval training (HIIT) has received a lot of attention lately, and rightly so. I've seen (and done) various forms of this type of exercise. If you're not familiar with it, HIIT means you work really hard for a period of time and then rest for a period of time. It truly is that simple. Imagine a graph that looks like a mountain range with high points and low points, which represents your work and heart rate during a HIIT workout. We will talk about HIIT a few times throughout this book, so I want you to know some of the reasons it's so great.

HIIT:

- Improves cardiorespiratory fitness.

- Increases insulin sensitivity, meaning it helps bring glucose to the muscles more effectively. We don't want excess glucose, or sugar, floating around our bloodstream otherwise it affects the pancreas's insulin production. Alternatively, it gets stored as adipose, otherwise known as body fat.

- Elevates "good" HDL cholesterol.

- Lowers blood pressure.

- Ignites the breakdown or burning of fat by the muscles you are exercising.[3]

If you've worked with a trainer or peeked at a gym fitness schedule, you've probably been exposed to HIIT. A quick search on YouTube offers more options than I have the time or energy to do. Most of these classes and videos I support. But the one caveat often forgotten? The harder the intensity of your workout, the shorter its duration should be. More is *not* more with HIIT. In fact, the opposite is true. The longer the duration, the less effort you are able to give, decreasing the overall metabolic benefits. If you are in a true high-intensity workout in which your effort is 90 percent, your body will not perform at that level for an hour.

Have you ever heard the term Tabata? Named after the Japanese researcher who created it, the Tabata style of HIIT involves working at maximum effort for twenty seconds and taking ten seconds off for a total of eight rounds. The total time of a Tabata set is four minutes. *Four minutes!* When combined with other natural movements, extensive research shows this is enough to achieve heart health. Like we discussed in Chapter 10, I do advise you to warm up and cool down appropriately so you don't injure yourself. We aren't fifteen anymore!

Dr. Len Kravitz, a leading exercise-science researcher, recommends HIIT workouts lasting from ten to twenty minutes as they are highly effective and time-efficient.[4]

If you're over forty, give yourself a minimum of forty-eight hours in between HIIT workouts and perform no more than three HIIT workouts a week. Rest is critical, which we will cover in Chapter 20: "No Rest for the Weary."

That awesome HIIT has a side effect: cortisol. However, despite what you may have heard about cortisol, it's not all bad. As author and fitness educator Pete McCall explains:

> *Cortisol is a catabolic steroid hormone produced by the adrenal gland in response to stress, low blood sugar, and exercise. It supports energy metabolism during long periods of exercise by facilitating the breakdown of triglyceride and protein to create the glucose necessary to help fuel exercise. Cortisol is released when the body experiences too much physical stress or is not sufficiently recovered from a previous workout. While cortisol helps promote fat metabolism, exercising for too long can elevate levels of cortisol to catabolize (break down) muscle protein for fuel instead of conserving it to be used to repair damaged tissues.*[5]

In layman's terms: Cortisol helps your body create energy to help fuel exercise. However, too much stress or exercise or not enough rest creates excess cortisol. Exercising for too long also releases cortisol, which can break down muscle protein for fuel instead of repairing damaged tissues.

Some cortisol is your friend. In fact, it's necessary for fuel regulation. But it's also an enemy if you have too much. A frenemy. Just like your long, intense exercise sessions.

Lose the long breaks in strength training to shorten your workouts

Next door to the classroom where I right stepped, left stepped in that thong leotard (*have I mentioned how awful those were?*) was the free-weight room. I could see through the windows on my way to my classroom and always wondered, "Are they even working in there?" Most of the time I saw muscular men sitting on a bench shooting the breeze.

Yes, they were working. Their hypertrophy-focused method involved lifting heavy weights to fatigue, then resting two to three minutes in between sets. I don't know how long they were in there because I never joined them. But a quick calculation of doing just ten different exercises three times each (with a three-minute break in between) tells me ninety minutes was not unusual. The part of me that thrives on efficiency could never do that.

Granted, my strength training goals are different than those men, and my strength training workouts require less time to achieve. My sets are all about efficiency. Either I only rest for thirty seconds in between sets or I alternate between upper-body and lower-body exercises. For example, twelve push-ups, twelve squats, and repeat two more times.

If you wonder if you'll feel the benefits of strength training in such a short time, you will. Just make sure you're choosing the right load (weight and reps). In thirty minutes you can work every major area of your body and still have time to make yourself some eggs before your day starts.

Increase your metabolism through NEAT, not long exercise sessions

"NEAT!" I'm not trying to use the vocabulary of a fresh-faced girl from the 1950s. NEAT is an acronym for non-exercise activity thermogenesis. It's a fancy way of describing movement that's not formal exercise. When you take the stairs, park farther away from your destination, and walk to your children's room to ask them a question rather than text, you are increasing your NEAT. What does this have to do with not working out an hour? Because NEAT provides a host of health benefits with a lot less sweat.

NEAT:

- Encourages your body to move more often, as we were intended.

- Increases your BMR, basal metabolic rate, or the amount of energy the body uses to support itself. Twenty lean non-exercisers burned an additional 350 calories per day above their obese counterparts by standing, walking, and fidgeting significantly more during the day.[6]

- Helps your body resist weight gain after weight loss.[7]

- Reduces mortality rate. A large (over 152,000 participants) seven-year study concluded that one to two hours of NEAT per day results in mortality reduction of 50–60 percent for women.[8] Even smaller amounts show great effects. Moving three minutes for every thirty minutes of sitting lowers mortality and combats the negative effects of sustained sitting.[9]

- Helps your body sustain LPL levels and maintain its ability to burn fat. Lipoprotein lipase (LPL) is an enzyme that plays a critical role in converting fat into energy.[10]

This is the best part about NEAT: There are no rules. You know I'm a huge fan of that. In order to increase your NEAT, simply start moving more. This includes walking. Yes, take walks and never underestimate the power and benefits of walking. You'll learn even more about the benefits of walking in the chapter "Walking Isn't a Real Workout."

Try these approaches to increase your NEAT:

- Walk more in your daily activities, and force yourself to walk farther distances.
- Leash up your dog and walk down the block and back.
- Take the stairs instead of the elevator.
- Work from home? Move your printer to the farthest point away you reasonably can.
- Walk upstairs to deliver the toilet paper rather than leaving it on the stair steps for your kids to grab.
- Park in the farthest spot away at church (bonus: this blesses others and gives newcomers the closer spaces).
- Walk to the mailbox rather than stopping on your drive home (yes, I'm guilty of this as well).

Small movement changes in your daily life may contribute to positive changes in your overall health and weight management goals. And isn't that our endgame anyway?

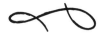

Truth be told, I still exercise a full hour every now and then. Most of the time that's because I have someone by my side and we are deep in conversation. It's how I best connect with my handful of regular walking friends. And I learned long ago, it sure treats my body better than lunch out or happy hour.

If you love moving for sixty minutes, go for it. If that's what makes you thrive and feel great, I applaud you. But if you are getting your hour of exercise in simply because that's what you've always done or feel unsuccessful if you don't, then let the information in this chapter give you the confidence to cut that time. Cut it in half, or even give it 16 percent (ten minutes). Something is better than nothing, and your "something" does not have to be an hour.

The Simple Take:
One hour of exercise simply is not necessary for
cardiovascular health or even weight management.
In fact, it may be that you are sabotaging your efforts
with your long, intense workout sessions. Get in
however much you can, and supplement that by
increasing your NEAT.

20-Minute HIIT

Now that I've (hopefully) convinced you of the benefits to shorter workouts, it's time to create our own! Following is a list of higher-intensity exercises.

Bodyweight with Impact

- Jump squats
- 180 jump squats
- Side-to-side squats
- Burbees
- Alternating jump lunges
- Jump rope

Lower Impact

- Bike
- Plank jacks
- Mountain climbers
- Squat thrusts
- Elliptical
- Rower
- Treadmill walk at high incline

Workout

Warm up for a minimum of five minutes, preferably ten. I've listed a few ideas below. When I do running sprints using the cardiovascular HIIT method, I take ten to fifteen minutes so I don't injure myself. Trust me: I learned the hard way when I jumped in too fast.

Warm-Up Ideas

- Brisk walk
- Indoor bicycle
- Light jacks
- Low kicks (start really low and gradually increase the height)
- Dynamic stretching (continuously moving through the stretch rather than holding it)

If you downloaded the resource guide, I've also provided a bonus ten-minute mobility warm-up flow.

TABATA STYLE
Bodyweight HIIT

Choose two exercises. Name them A and B. A true tabata set is :20 seconds of the highest intensity possible followed by a :10 second break for eight rounds. Perform any of the following combinations from the list above. Start with the first combination (ABABABAB) and progress to the last (AAAAAAAA).

- A B A B A B A B
- A A B B A A B B
- A A A A B B B B
- A A A A A A A A

Cardiovascular HIIT

Choose any of the following movements. Perform for :20 seconds and break :40. Repeat. Start with 10 sets, working your way up to no more than 20.

- Run
- Bike (stationary or outdoors)
- Swim
- Elliptical
- Walk at high incline

Note: If you are using indoor cardio equipment, it can take a few seconds to ramp the equipment up to full speed. Factor this in to your :20 second interval. Consider starting a few seconds early to reap full benefits of the :20 second interval. If you're using a treadmill, simply straddle the treadmill during the rest time rather than adjusting the speed and/or incline.

Cooldown

Cool down for several minutes to bring your heart rate down. Stopping a workout without safely taking your heart down with it can result in blood pooling in your extremities, which can lead to clots. No thank you to that. Use any of the following to cool down:

- Walk
- Indoor bicycle
- Stretching the muscles you just used
- Light yoga, like sun salutations
- If you downloaded the resource guide, I've also provided a bonus ten-minute mobility cooldown flow.

CHAPTER FIFTEEN

No pain, no gain

Of all the rules we break in this book, this might be my favorite. Or least favorite, I suppose. I see this slogan all over the place. On T-shirts. Memes. Pinterest. Gyms. It's the one chapter example most people resonated with when I told them the premise of this book. It seems like everyone has heard or seen the slogan "No pain, no gain."

"No pain, no gain" is an adage that to make progress or to be successful, one must suffer. This suffering may be in a physical or mental sense.

We're probably all too familiar with this phrase. Its roots go back to the second century and have ties to Benjamin Franklin and Jane Fonda (perhaps the only time those two have been tied together). In my mind, it's used in a weathered Gold's Gym with some burly gray-haired man coaching a young boxer. He's yelling at an impressionable whippersnapper who is looking for a way out of his situation or perhaps trying to deal with his emotions in a boxing ring.

Maybe that saying worked for that kid, but it's not meant for me. I don't want pain. The thought of it certainly doesn't motivate me.

Merriam-Webster.com defines pain as "a localized or generalized *unpleasant* bodily sensation or complex of sensations that causes mild to *severe physical discomfort* and *emotional distress* and typically results from *bodily disorder* (such as injury or disease)."[1]

Unpleasant.

Severe physical discomfort.

Emotional distress.

Bodily disorder.

Call me crazy, but none of these seem to jive with the same dictionary's definition of health: "the condition of being sound in body, mind, or spirit; a condition in which someone or something is thriving or doing well."[2]

Most of my clients are around my age, give or take ten years. While we still feel twenty-eight in some ways and want to move as such, in actuality we are not. I try my best to develop class and training structure so it's challenging but not impossible. As with any trainer worth the value of her sports bra (which, by the way, are not cheap), I individualize and meet my clients where they are.

In my tight-knit classes, I've learned to read my clients' faces. My quiet introvert will just sigh, and I know she's struggling but pressing on. My fierce runner loves challenges, but sometimes the workout threatens her resolve. And my client who has had so many surgeries she seems half-bionic just keeps fighting. Her steel-faced focus gives her away, though, when she's pushing through.

Because I love these women and they know it, I lightly poke fun at their faces. I'd like to believe they are fine with it. But then I'll turn serious and ask three words: "Hurt or hard?" In other words, I want to know if they are in pain or just momentarily challenged.

Is exercising hard? Yes. Will there be times you find yourself gritting your teeth to finish out those last few seconds of a tough movement? Of course. But should that be painful? Absolutely not.

The older I get, the better I am at listening to my body. Always responding to it? That's a different story. My back starts to twinge. My feet feel prickly in the morning. My shoulder asks for a self-massage. What do I do? I'm embarrassed to admit I ignore them sometimes. Being a fitness professional guarantees I can avoid injury if I know the nuts and bolts of my body, right? Ahem. Not so much. I think I'm better than these signs; I know more. Unfortunately, ignoring isn't effective with my shoulder, and it's not with my body either. These twinges eventually cry out louder, waking me up in the middle of the night until they finally morph into an all-out revolt.

You've probably heard the modern definition of insanity: doing the same thing over and over again but expecting different results. (In fact, this is not a definition. While I like the concept of it, Merriam-Webster holds no such explanation.)

Those prickling needles in my heel first thing in the morning will not go away if I keep lacing up my running shoes five days a week. My back will remain tight as long as I am bending over my computer or phone. If I keep doing what I'm doing, I can't expect something to change. My insanity causes pain.

Hurt is experiencing pain. Hurt is an unfamiliar twinge that doesn't feel right, or perhaps an acute irritation. Hurt might flare up an old injury or, heaven forbid, create a new one. Hurt is not okay. It's my body's way of communicating. It might be saying I am working one muscle too much, or I need to strengthen a different one. It may even be saying I need to rest and not work.

What's a gal to do when the pain comes knocking? Please don't follow my lead and ignore it. Instead, try these three options:

1. *Rest.* Yes, you heard that correctly. Rest in various forms. Our body heals and repairs itself while sleeping, so get a few extra zzz's at night. If possible, take a catnap. Once you're getting enough shut-eye, how can you rest your body while you're awake? Gently moving the afflicted area helps encourage blood flow, which carries healing nutrients. Gentle is the operative word, though. We will talk more about rest in Chapter 20.

2. *Move differently.* If you find yourself in pain from walking, try biking. Knees bugging you from squats? Try focusing on strengthening your upper body for a bit. Our body is meant to move in all directions; try to find a new way of moving it. Not sure how to move differently? Find a mobility class, or download the mobility resource referenced in "There's One Right

Way to Exercise," which guarantees you'll move in different directions.

3. *See a professional.* Sometimes pain is our body's way of saying there's a serious issue that needs to be addressed. Do not ignore these signals if they last or get progressively worse. Thank goodness we have a variety of professionals who can help. From orthopedic surgeons to physical therapists to acupuncturists to myofascial release specialists, there is likely someone who can assist you. They may even be able to heal you.

What about preventing pain? Points one and two above are a great place to start. Resting and moving your body differently are great injury preventers. I've also found gentle foam rolling to be helpful (this chapter's resource includes the basics of foam rolling). Also, don't ignore those tweaks and twinges. That's your body communicating with you.

Once we've got hurt taken care of, we can address hard. Hard is an opportunity. It's a choice. Do we push through or stop short of what we can do? It's recognizing the current limits of our body and choosing to raise the bar just a little bit. Maybe we pick up the speed, jump an inch higher, or increase our dumbbells. Meeting Hard and staring her in the face can take your physical fitness to the next level.

Sometimes you meet Hard and find yourself sore the next day. You might feel yesterday's squats when you walk up the stairs or feel some tenderness in your chest from push-ups. This is not pain. This is Hard reminding you of your work. Hard is good. Hard is sometimes an internal fight to gain strength, endurance, or even flexibility.

But here's something else you may not hear often from fitness professionals: you don't have to challenge Hard every time. You can simply acknowledge her and proclaim, "Not today." Not every day is meant to spar with Hard. She can show up at inopportune times.

She doesn't know if you're coming off a cold, if you were up all night with a sick child, or if work is so stressful you don't have time to eat. Hard sometimes shows up when we need her baby sister, Enough, instead.

I have several friends who grew up as the family caboose, the last of several children. As adults, they are agreeable and gregarious. Sometimes they tell stories of their youth when they simply followed their older siblings around. They played whatever game their big sister directed and did so happily. Being included was Enough.

Enough is just happy you're working out with her. She may not need to achieve a personal best today. Enough is glad to be doing something. Just like we talked about in the last chapter, something is better than nothing.

Enough can show up in various ways:

- Walking when you were supposed to go on a run.
- Performing an entire workout at a low-impact level when the instructor seems to be jumping four feet off the ground.
- Choosing a stress-reducing gentle yoga class instead of the scheduled boxing class.
- Focusing on increasing NEAT (nonexercise movement) rather than actually exercising (we discussed NEAT in the last chapter).

Enough has an important place in our health. She's happy to be in our presence and provides more benefits than we give her credit for. Enough gives us grace when we just don't have it in us.

I've hung out with Enough for varying amounts of time: a day, a week, a full season. During the 2020 summer of COVID-19, I trained clients outdoors upwards of twelve hours a week. I coached, demonstrated movements, and joined in the last twenty seconds of a set in the hopes of energizing my clients. All of this I executed in Houston's oppressive heat and humidity, where it is difficult to simply exist outside during summer, much less exercise. After two days of trying to get my own workout in before my clients, I threw in the towel. No more personal workouts. This summer would not be the strongest one ever but one of being active without intentional exercise. It was the summer of Enough. This attitude worked fine. Eventually, though, I got tired of Enough. She didn't offer much physical or mental stimulation. By September, I found myself ready for the fitness goals, plans, and structures in which I thrive.

Enough faded away for the season, though she occasionally showed up. Like that little sister, I endured her for a day or two, then sent her on her way. She's worth the place in my workouts at the appropriate time. Other times, Hard takes the lead.

There's a time to invite and welcome Hard, who will make you stronger, faster, or feel more accomplished. There's a time when Enough is just that. Hard is good. Enough is good. Hurt...not good. And Hurt is pain. No pain is good. Find your gains in Hard, and don't invite Hurt in the door when she comes knocking. No pain, no gain, no thanks.

The Simple Take:
Pain is not an accomplishment or a badge of honor.
It's your body's way of communicating with you that
something isn't right. Take preventative measures like
resting, moving your body differently, and inviting
Enough in every now and then.

Foam Rolling

Foam Rolling is an underappreciated method of preventing and healing pain. Access the video in the resource guide for a demo focusing on several common tight areas. If you're already familiar with how to roll, add these into your routine as a warm-up or cooldown.

- Iliotibial (IT) bands (on the outside of your thighs)
- Adductors (inner thighs)
- Gastrocnemius (calf muscles)
- Glutes
- Latissimus dorsi (lats—large flat muscles on either side of your back)

CHAPTER SIXTEEN

Pass the bucket

A friend once invited me to an indoor cycling class during the height of its popularity. Indoor cycling is also known by a name synonymous with twirling, but that name is trademarked. I choose not to be taken to court, so I will hereby refer to it as indoor cycling. It's worth noting that during this time I was teaching group fitness classes, but I had not yet tried indoor cycling. It's also worth noting that I would go on to lead this type of class in the future.

At zero dark thirty in the morning, my friend and I arrived a few minutes early to class, where she helped me get situated on a stationary bike. My feet lacked the fancy shoes that clipped into the pedals that the other participants wore. Even a greater travesty: my rear was covered in simple shorts, rather than padded compression shorts or even leggings. I paid for that later in the day as I waddled around with chafed inner thighs and feeling like my sit bones were bruised.

During class, I followed the instructor's guidance. Sometimes we increased the resistance and simulated a climb, while other times we decreased the resistance and tried to achieve maximum rotations per minute. In the most brutal of songs, we did both. Cue the pool of sweat on the floor. But as a new student, I was still getting the hang of what all the terminology meant: "Increase your resistance to an eight." "We're going for a hard climb." "I want your intensity at a nine." *Huh?*

Never mind I felt a little like a hamster in a stationary wheel. My confusion kept me from fully experiencing the class, but trust me: I still worked hard.

Following the final cooldown and stretching, my friend looked at me and said with a smile, "That was awesome. I almost threw up." Dang it, I didn't almost throw up! Does that mean I didn't work hard enough? Also: *What? Was I supposed to throw up? Is that the secret indoor cycling goal no one told me about?*

Lest indoor cycling feel picked upon, I've heard other stories of gyms strategically placing buckets near stations where people might need to spontaneously eject the contents of their stomach. Heck, I've seen my own son finish a tough lap around the track and immediately hover over the trash can.

But still: When did this become the litmus test? Why is it a good thing if our body is thrown into a point of revulsion? If I threw up after any other beneficial activity, I'd be concerned. Running to the bathroom in the middle of eating a spinach salad would not cause me to think, "Oh, this salad is extra good!" Not once has a good prayer session with God caused me to vomit—even when I read in Proverbs 26:11 about a dog returning to his vomit (so a fool repeats his folly).

Every four years, I gleefully anticipate the summer Olympics. I especially appreciate those events in which I've participated as a recreational athlete. Watching Katie Ledecky complete 400 meters across the pool in three minutes fifty-six seconds is even more impressive when I compare it to my seven-ish minutes from a triathlon several years ago. And while I never formally ran track, I've done enough laps around that big four hundred meter loop to stand in awe and wonder at Allyson Felix's forty-nine seconds.

Never, not even once, have I witnessed any of these athletes complete their event, place their hands on their knees, and empty the contents of their preworkout meal. You don't see trash cans at the end of a race at the professional level. Granted, every now and then I hear about that happening prior to an event, but that's often (understandably) tied to nerves. If it's not normal for the highest-caliber athletes to throw up after their workouts, why do we think this is okay for us?

It's not. This behavior is often the result of an imbalance, either physiologically or psychologically. It's your body's way of providing a stress response. It is no surprise to anyone that imbalance is the antithesis of what I strive for. What kind of lopsidedness, you ask? Assuming you have no medical issues, consider one of these potential culprits of your pre- or postworkout sickness.

Hydration

My son's club track practice used to begin at 5:00 p.m. after a full day of school. When the season began, he had a rough go of reconditioning himself. After a few weeks, however, he found his rhythm. Most practices left him feeling strong, and his times decreased. During practices over Christmas break, however, I found myself confused when he reverted back to getting sick after hard sets, especially since he was getting more sleep and the weather was cooler.

Before making an appointment with a gastroenterologist (which I do believe is necessary sometimes), I asked Dr. Google. Several times I noticed hydration mentioned. He may have been sleeping more, but because his schedule was off, so was his water intake. We began focusing on making sure he drank plenty of fluids upon awakening as well as throughout the day. Poof! Problem solved.

He's not alone. According to the National Institutes of Health, "nausea and vomiting are relatively frequent GI symptoms in athletes, especially those performing endurance sport disciplines. In the majority of the cases, they are particular physiological reactions to strenuous exercise and *might be alleviated by proper hydration*."[1]

How do you know if hydration is an issue? My first recommendation is to pay attention to your water consumption throughout the day. Aim for at least sixty-four ounces, but if you are outside or sweating a lot, you may need more. A good way to know if you're intaking enough is to pay attention to your output. Your urine indicates your hydration levels. The darker your urine, the more dehydrated you are. Shoot for a lemonade-colored or lighter urine.

If you are an excessive sweater (like I am), consider weighing yourself naked before and after a tough workout. Losing more than 2 percent of our body weight during exercise can have a detrimental effect on the body, such as a slowed delivery of nutrients and oxygen to cells, altered body temperature, muscle cramping, decreased cognitive function, and more, all of which can affect gastrointestinal symptoms.[2]

The good news about vomiting due to low hydration is this is a relatively easy fix. Increase your water (preferably hours before your workout) and see if everything stays down.

Electrolyte levels

Electrolytes are positively or negatively charged ions that conduct electrical activity. In the human body, the right concentration of electrolytes is necessary to maintain fluid balance, muscle contraction, and neural activity. The kidneys work to maintain electrolyte balance by conserving or excreting electrolytes. Water follows the movement of electrolytes, particularly sodium and chloride, meaning that water is drawn to locations where electrolytes are most concentrated. Therefore, electrolytes play a critical role in maintaining the equilibrium of water throughout the body, particularly during exercise when electrolytes and water can be lost through sweating.[3]

Significant electrolytes include sodium, potassium, and chloride along with magnesium, calcium, phosphate, and bicarbonates. Electrolytes come from our food and fluids.[4]

If you're having terrible flashbacks to high school chemistry, I understand. Basically, *electrolytes provide fluid balance so your body's systems can optimally run*. Because water follows the electrolytes, it's important you have the Goldilocks amount...not too little, not too much.

The tricky part in maintaining this balance is when we begin to sweat excessively. Some electrolytes, like sodium and chloride, are lost in higher concentrations through sweat, while others, like potassium, magnesium, and calcium, are lost in lower concentrations. If you've ever discovered a white line on your black sports bra after a hard workout, you can assume you are a salty sweater. (Me too. This also happens on my hats, so much that I only purchase hats I can throw in the washing machine after a hot session.)

What does this have to do with wanting to throw up? We get nauseous when our electrolytes are out of balance. And chances are, you may not be getting enough electrolytes in general. Many Americans underconsume vitamins, including electrolytes like potassium, magnesium, and calcium.[5] Not surprisingly, we get more than enough of the electrolyte sodium, as we tend to overconsume that from our processed food.

If you're drinking plenty of water but still needing that bucket, consider your electrolytes. Increase your potassium by consuming foods like bananas, dried apricots, spinach, sweet potatoes, and avocados. Magnesium-rich foods include wheat bran; cooked spinach; Brazil nuts; cashews; seeds like flax, sunflower, and pumpkin; quinoa; and—wait for it—dark chocolate. (I'm doing a little happy dance here.)

Food timing

I can literally eat a couple of fried eggs and then go for a run. In fact, this used to be my prerun standard breakfast. I also realize I'm more the exception than the norm. If you find you're getting sick or feeling nauseous after a particular type of food or after a certain amount of time after eating, it's time to do some investigative work. Just like we talked about experimenting in "Go All In and Do It Right," play around with not only what you eat but also when you eat it. In general, the closer to your workout, the more carbs you want because they are easier to digest. Higher-fat foods should be consumed a few hours prior to exercise. If you need a little something in your stomach right before a workout, try a little peanut butter on a banana (with a potassium bonus!). But it's really up to you to figure out what fuels you best. After all, those fried eggs (which are not lowfat) treat me well on long runs.

Mindset

Now that we've discussed all the science-y things, let's get to the heart of the matter. Are you actually *wanting* to work out so hard that you throw up?

Sometimes, feeling ill after a workout is actually a goal: "That was awesome. I almost threw up." This isn't always the case, of course. Getting sick can be attributed to more-scientific issues as listed above. But somewhere along the line, we've convinced ourselves we need to deplete every bit of energy before checking off the workout box. Sure, sometimes that happens. But every time? No ma'am, no thank you.

If your trainer is sporting a tank top reading "Pass the Bucket," I encourage you to think about his goals for you. Do you want to trust your body with someone who is literally trying to make you sick? To be fair, buckets on the gym floor obviously don't mean that's his goal for you. It may simply be preventative measures for the twenty-five-year-old weekend warriors after a hard Friday night (speaking of electrolyte imbalance). I don't fault or blame trying to contain a potential mess. But if your trainer puffs out his chest at the beginning of your session and proudly predicts you'll be meeting the bucket, think long and hard about that relationship and if he truly wants what's best for you.

What about the trainer in your head? The one yelling "harder, faster, more more more!" What does she want for you? Is she punishing you for eating something...not exercising enough...your tight-fitting pants? That's another relationship worth severing. She doesn't have your long-term health in mind. Perhaps she doesn't even care how you feel a few hours from now when everyone is playing in the pool but your headache prevents you from joining them. She only wants short-term results, like burning as many calories as possible with no lasting consequence.

It might be time to fire that trainer. Look for a new one with a different approach. One who gently reminds you to hydrate. She allows mistakes in food timing but learns from those mistakes. Ideally, find one whose name is Grace. She knows not every workout is going to be fantastic, and she allows that. She is gentle. Encouraging. Forgiving. She wants you to work hard, but she allows rest days.

Yes, getting sick during or after a workout happens. There's no shame in this, and the reason can be as simple as needing to drink more water earlier in the day or less right before you begin exercising. But equating that with a successful workout? I beg to differ. Lose the bucket and find some Grace.

The Simple Take:
If you find yourself consistently throwing up during
or after a workout, make sure you are hydrated and
have consumed electrolyte-rich foods. And make sure
vomiting isn't the goal of you or your trainer.

Track-Meet Smoothie *and* Check-the-Boxes Chia Pudding

Here are two electrolyte-rich recipes to keep you balanced.

Track-Meet Smoothie

Regardless of the sport, if your child is an outdoor athlete, you both have experienced sweat dripping down your back while waiting to play or watch. I created this for my son when he ran club track. Nothing says hot like a Houston summer track meet. His events often bookended the meets, which meant he had six to eight hours in between running. Even if he sat under the tent and played on his phone, he was still sweating out precious fluids and electrolytes needed to perform well.

As we've learned, low electrolyte levels can cause stomach distress. Use this when you need to increase your potassium and fluid intake.

One note: This is not a protein shake. This carb-o-licious smoothie offers plenty of electrolytes to replenish fluids lost in sweat. It's easily absorbed and is a good complement to drinking plenty of water. If you or your athlete is not consuming right before their sporting event, I recommend pairing with a light protein snack like string cheese, turkey, or nuts to prevent blood-sugar spikes (and consequent crashes).

Ingredients

- 1 16-oz. bottle coconut water
- ½ cup frozen strawberries
- ½ cup frozen pineapple
- Orange juice or more coconut water to thin if desired

Serves 2. If making in a single-serve blender, halve the recipe.

Directions

Blend ingredients in your preferred mixer (I love my Magic Bullet). Use more or less coconut water depending on your desired consistency. Transfer to a double-walled stainless-steel water bottle if transporting to a summer track meet (or any hot outdoor event).

Check-the-Boxes Chia Pudding

If you find yourself needing the bucket during a workout, this is an electrolyte-rich snack to help balance your magnesium levels. Just make sure to enjoy it several hours before exercising, as the high fiber content could have you running to the bathroom instead of the bucket if your digestive system isn't acclimated to it.

The recipe below is a curation of foods containing magnesium. You'll get added benefits of Omega-3s, calcium, and potassium as well. Make sure you use cacao powder as opposed to cocoa powder for maximum magnesium benefits. By consuming this snack, check off a significant portion of your recommended daily allowances for all of these nutrients.

And a bonus! You'll check off several other nutritional boxes as well. With this snack, you'll receive twelve grams of fiber, which is half of the recommended amount for women over forty. Enjoying this chia pudding will get you well on your way to checking off your fiber goal for the day. When made with 2 percent milk, you'll also receive almost ten grams of protein.

In a 12-oz. glass jar, combine the following:

- ½ cup milk, your choice
- 2 tbs. chia seeds
- 1 tbs. cacao powder
- ½ banana, well mashed
- ½ tsp. ground cinnamon
- ½ tsp. honey (optional)

Place the lid on the glass jar. Shake until well blended. Refrigerate at least one hour. Stir and enjoy. May prepare up to three days in advance.

CHAPTER SEVENTEEN

Walking isn't a real workout

*M*y husband sometimes feels decades older than he is. Because of his psoriatic arthritis, he experiences seasons of inflammation and flare-ups. This is common in rheumatoid arthritis sufferers, but symptoms vary. He may experience spine pain, tenderness, and swelling in his fingers, or overall aches. Listing them all sounds like a pharmaceutical advertisement disclaimer. Compounding the issue is his age and the inflammation's tendency to cause more injury. When something gets wounded, we are never quite sure if it's his arthritis, muscles, or joints trying to tell us something. It's a guessing game full of experiments.

In one such season, he decided to completely pause working out his upper body, hoping to heal a six-month-long shoulder injury. "Didn't he go to the doctor?" you ask. He's a man. So, no. But he did desire to stay active, which I admired.

One Sunday, he joined me on a walk. While we were discussing his workout options, he dismissed walking.

"Sure, I'll walk. But what's this doing for me anyway?"

Again, keep in mind he's a dude. His goals are different. Let's be honest: while women are generally trained to take up as *little* space as possible, men are trained to take up as *much* space as possible. In the words of my kids, they want to get "jacked." If you want proof, talk to any teen boy about what muscle groups he focuses on. Chest and biceps, or biceps and chest. They want as much mass in those areas as possible. While it's easy for me to dismiss my husband's desire to remain defined, I have to understand this desire has been conditioned in him almost as long as I've been wanting six-pack abs. Walking, unfortunately, doesn't do much for the chest and biceps.

"What does walking do for me anyway?" sat with me. I paused, not sure how to answer. As the resident nerd in my house, I tend to be overbearing when it comes to health education. "Well, do you want my trainer's perspective?"

I don't know if the "sure" he provided indicated true interest or that he was simply humoring me. Regardless, I found it to be an opportunity to educate him on one of the most underappreciated forms of exercise.

Why, exactly, is walking so underrated? I think it's because it's not very interesting. After all, it's our primary means of leaving point A and arriving at point B. If it is so good for us, why is it so easy to do? Maybe, just maybe, because we were *meant to walk more*.

We used to walk more than we do now. Jesus and His disciples traveled miles in between cities. Women walked to the well to gather water for the day. But as our ability to see our world expanded to planes, trains, and automobiles, we sat more. Computers and smartphones revolutionized the way we live. Now, rather than walking to my boys' rooms to tell them dinner is ready, I text them. I am not proud of this by the way.

Yet walking remains an integral part of our lives. Yes, it is our primary means of traversing short distances. But it also reflects who we are: what is important to us, what life stage we are in, and what we value.

We've used walking for:

- Raising awareness for causes dear to our heart
- Hiking through God's creations
- Lulling babies to sleep
- Connecting with friends
- Making our way to the blessed coffeepot in the morning
- Following our children up and down the sidelines during their sports events
- Completing household chores

This incomplete list demonstrates how essential walking is in our everyday lives. Maybe that's why it doesn't seem like a big deal to get out there and do it for exercise. But make no mistake, walking is beneficial to your health.

Walking actually is worth your time, possibly in ways you haven't considered.

Core strength

A quick lesson on your core: it's much more than those six-pack abs I'm conditioned to desire. It's a combination of twenty muscle groups[1] that work together to stabilize movement and protect your organs. Think of a corset running from just below your bra line to just below your rear. Men can envision their core beginning right under their pectorals. Pretty much every muscle in that region is part of your core. Your core is not one muscle but a region that controls the motion of our pelvis, femurs, rib cage, and spine.

When I speak to potential clients about their goals, they often include "core strengthening." Fair enough. I add this to our programming, challenging the full gamut of these twenty muscles, either directly or indirectly. Another way? Throw on your shoes and hit the sidewalk. While you're walking, roll your shoulders back, pull your rib cage together (I also use the term "lace" your ribcage together), and gently pull your belly button to your spine. If you're not sure what this means, imagine you knew someone was going to punch you in the gut (I hope this never happens by the way). You would tighten everything up to protect your insides. This is essentially engaging your core. Keep your ears in line with your shoulders. If you need a visual refresher, remember I've provided a demo video of this in "Jump In and Get 'Er Done." Be aware of your posture as you move and walk. I hunch over if I'm not careful.

Every time your foot makes contact with the ground, your body is accelerated downward by the force of gravity. At the same time, the ground exerts an equal and opposite force upwards into your lower leg, called ground reaction force (GRF); these two competing forces intersect around the body's center of gravity.[2] In layman's terms, this means that simply by walking, you are utilizing the muscles that support your center of gravity: your core. Yes, I can share a million other beneficial core-strengthening exercises, but walking gives you the foundation to perform them when you use proper posture.

Cardiovascular health

We tend to think because we aren't breathing hard when we walk that our heart isn't reaping benefits. At least I think this. (This is another absurd rule that does not have its own chapter but deserves recognition.) The reality is that walking provides just as many benefits to lowering my risk of cardiovascular disease as running. A 2013 study of nearly 50,000 people tested whether walking and running provided equivalent health benefits. When the same amount of energy was expended, the walkers had a risk level 9 percent lower than those who were inactive. The runners? 4.5 percent.[3] Walkers reduced their heart disease risk more than runners when they burned the same amount of calories. Keep in mind this study assumes equal energy expenditure, or calories burned, so you'll have to walk farther to make it equal to the distance you'd cover running. In other words, walk four miles or run four miles to burn the same amount of energy. The walk will take longer, but you'll get greater heart disease risk benefits. Regardless, walk with confidence knowing you're taking care of your heart.

Energy bump

Going for a walk when tired can increase oxygen flow throughout the body. It can increase the number of mitochondria, the portion of the muscle cells that converts oxygen to energy. More mitochondria means your body becomes more efficient at converting oxygen to energy. Going for a walk when tired can also increase the hormones responsible for elevating energy levels.[4] If you're like me and those science-y words make you feel a little cross-eyed, here's your take-away: walking wakes you up. Even just a few minutes can achieve this result.

Mood booster

You've probably heard of a "runner's high." Perhaps you have experienced it. We receive endorphins with exercise. These endorphins give us feelings of exhilaration, reduced stress, and/or euphoria. The good news is you don't need to actually run to achieve a runner's high. Simply exercise at a moderate level for twenty minutes or more[5] and you can join that runner's high club (not to be confused with the mile high club).

Not to pile on the pitfalls of aging, but as we age we lose dopamine, the "happy hormone" that provides pleasure rewards. In fact, with each passing decade, we lose up to 13 percent of the dopamine receptors in the reward system.[6] Walking, and all physical activity, helps prevent that decline by releasing dopamine.

Regular physical activity modifies the default state of the nervous system so that it becomes more balanced and less prone to fight, flight, or fright.[7] We handle stress better with a balanced nervous system. Got a challenge to work through in a relationship? Try tackling it on the sidewalks or trail rather than the couch. I can give personal testimony to this one—it works!

Whether you're in a short-term funk or have a history of depression, walking can be included as part of your mental health. And if it's not enough, remember to enlist the help of a counselor.

Arthritic support

Low-impact exercise increases blood flow to cartilage, which helps cartilage get the nutrients it needs to cushion and protect the ends of bones in your joints. Plus, any movement helps lubricate your joints, which decreases pain and stiffness and increases range of motion.[7] Obviously, this is a specific need for my husband. It's also something I'm acutely aware of with each passing year. What better way to combat arthritis than before it strikes?

Fresh-air benefits

I don't need research to know that fresh air is good for me. Even in the thick Houston summer, I feel better after getting outside for a minute. Sure, the humidity makes it feel like I'm swimming rather than walking, but I can't ignore the uplift. When my mind is jumbled, frenetic, or overfilled with emotions, even just a few minutes outside help. I take a few deep breaths and I can feel the intensity in my brain lower to a more manageable level. If you're in a harsh climate, find the best time of day to exercise outside. I like to go before the sun comes up, but I see plenty of walkers and runners getting their fresh air and exercise after sunset.

Blood pressure reduction

I've shared my blood pressure challenges, so this one is understandably close to my heart (no pun intended). Walking can help manage your blood pressure and is recommended by the American Heart Association. And if high blood pressure is something you fight, try to get as many steps in throughout the day as you can (even if it's just in your NEAT). One study showed that adults ages twenty to sixty-five who walked ten thousand steps per day for six months showed blood pressure improvement, with the systolic (top number) dropping by 5.57 points and the diastolic (bottom number) by 4.03 points.[8]

Low-impact option

I have clients with bad knees, bad hips, and bad backs. Sometimes my own knees, hips, and back need some TLC. We work through those issues and aim to strengthen them. But sometimes we still just need low-impact options. Walking is a great low-impact alternative. Have you been walking so long you don't feel it's challenging? Find some hills and utilize those. Add a weighted vest. Or increase your treadmill incline to a 6 percent incline or more. By adding these little challenges, your body can burn almost as many calories as running at a ten-minute running pace (or running at six miles per hour).[9]

You can even play around with speed walking for a few minutes before returning to your natural pace. Having lived at sea level for the past sixteen years, I forget you may have natural hills right outside your door. If so, hooray! Use these to challenge your core, heart, and lungs.

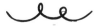

If you're hesitant about counting a walk as a workout, trust me: It actually is worth your time. It's a staple in my own workouts and is one of the greatest contributing factors to fostering my friendships and my mental health. And my body just feels good after this workout. Don't discount how beneficial walking can be to you.

The Simple Take:
Walking is most certainly a real workout. It can strengthen your core, heart, and mood and give you lower impact options for your changing body.

Do you love a long weekend walk? Then tune into the playlist I made just for you, full of upbeat, motivating songs. Find it on Spotify at "Your Worthy Body Walks." If you'd like some backstory to some of the songs I chose, tune into the "Graced Health" podcast episode titled "The Untold Stories Behind 'Your Worthy Body Walks Playlist' on Spotify." Find it in Season 12.

CHAPTER EIGHTEEN

There's one right way to exercise

"*A*re you still counting weight?" I asked my brother-in-law. The last time I saw him, he described this style of weight lifting. No, counting weight is not tallying the pounds added or even subtracted from the scale. It's aimed to lift a total amount of pounds during a workout. It's a mathematician's dream.

For example, the goal may be to lift 20,000 pounds in sixty minutes. This does not mean load up 20,000 pounds on a barbell and chest-press one time (though that would be impressive...also, impossible). Instead, the weight lifter totals the pounds lifted in a workout. Bench-pressing 200 pounds ten times accumulates 2,000 pounds. Eight reps of a squat with a 180-pound rack adds another 1,440 pounds. It turns into a game. Each one-hour workout is strategically designed to maximize reps and weight. My desire to actually do this type of workout is as high as getting a mammogram, but it is still interesting to me.

"Oh," he snorted, waving his hand. "That was like five or six programs ago. I tend to do something for about three months, then I get bored and move on to something else."

Some may call that quitting. I disagree. I like his way of thinking. It's the opposite of one of my new favorite words: fetishize.

According to MerriamWebster.com, *fetishize* is "to make a fetish of,"[1] and a *fetish* is "an object of irrational reverence or obsessive devotion."[2]

I thought this was a made-up word I heard on a fitness podcast until the dictionary proved otherwise. I have both participated in and witnessed the fetishizing of various health trends: indoor cycling, keto diets, HIIT, and low-carb diets, for example. None are inherently a problem. If indoor cycling is the ticket to get someone literally back in the saddle to regain their health, then I would do anything short of hanging streamers and tying balloons on their bike to celebrate.

I'm guilty of fetishizing as well. Recently I discovered mobility training, which involves increasing the range of motion of our joints. One of my favorite movements involves lying on the floor with one knee bent and twisted over the other. I take my arms in a "T" position on the floor, then drag my top arm along the floor from one side to the other in an arc. I call these Rainbow Arms, as the top arm makes the shape of a rainbow. The goal is to keep both the knee and top arm on the ground as I make this rainbow. I feel a fantastic stretch in my upper chest, and my humerus bone (upper arm) utilizes a full range of motion in the shoulder's ball-and-socket joint.

I liked this movement so much upon discovering it that I incorporated it into every client and class. Twelve times a week, we ended our time performing Rainbow Arms. I fetishized it. And then I sustained an overuse injury. Ironic, huh? Just because a movement is beneficial doesn't mean it's helpful to do all the time. I took a perfectly good movement, created an obsessive devotion, and ended up hurting myself.

When we take one particular mode of exercising and perform it over and over, we risk injuring ourselves. This is why good half-marathon training plans always include cross-training days, or exercise days other than running. As a side note, any good running plan should have this. It's not to overwhelm you. It's to keep you moving in different directions and to prevent injury. Trust it.

But we tend to hear about the latest workout program and think that's the only way to move. Or we find something we love and keep going back for more. You actually can have too much of a good thing that you enjoy. It's like me in the pantry. One piece of dark chocolate is fine. Ten is not.

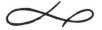

There's something exciting about starting a new workout routine. Part of my back-to-school planning includes writing out my weekly workouts. Changing up routines keeps it fresh and allows us to try new modalities. I claim to have exercise ADD during my own workouts, where I don't like doing anything for long periods of time. I learned I can't always coach this way, however. Asking twenty teen girls to change their movement every thirty seconds felt as frenetic as herding cats.

Changing up movements and workouts is scientifically based and even has a name: periodization. *Periodization* is dividing a training program into smaller stages, often intentionally changing workouts after an established period. Tony Horton and his P90X program took this mainstream by calling it "muscle confusion." The concept is the same: change your workouts after a particular amount of time for greater efficacy. Also for less boredom. This is probably why it fits me and my exercise ADD so well.

Technically, trainers can take programming into various stages and planning, focusing on cycles. These are lumped into two categories:

- *Nonlinear periodization* involves varying your workouts within the same week (this is my personal approach). For example, you might kick off Monday with a HIIT workout, strength train Tuesday and Thursday, do mobility or yoga on Wednesday, do another HIIT on Friday, and walk with a friend on Saturday. This type of workout schedule allows for varying levels of training stress. Sunday is a pure rest day, and Wednesday is for restorative lower-intensity workouts. Less stress = less chance of injury.

- *Linear periodization* focuses on a broader goal with macro (annual), meso (monthly), and micro (weekly) cycles. The half-marathon training programs I follow fall under this category.

Whatever the category, we trainers plan all kinds of geeky workouts and programs, building and shifting within the cycles. We follow the personal training book and what educators say is the most effective program. If you're a planner, do a little research into periodization training and go for it.

For the rest of us, here's a good rule of thumb: follow the four seasons, or at least the four seasons normal areas have. You may need to look beyond your climate and observe the traditional seasons. Here in the Houston area, we experience summer for seven sticky months, fall for eight days, "winter" (otherwise known as fall in other parts of the world) for three months, and some kind of combination of the three for the remainder of the time. If you don't have seasons, pretend you do. Every three months, change your movement.

Moving our bodies in different ways protects them. Just as your day-to-day life requires you to move in different ways, so should your workouts. On any given day, I'm loading a forty-eight pack of water into my cart, balancing on one foot while reaching up to get the stored stash of paper towels (why my people choose to store these on the top shelf is beyond me), or crouching down to reach for the dog bone under the couch.

Periodization offers science-backed support, specifically in strength/resistance training programs.[3] Read on for the high-level benefits.

Efficiency

Our bodies were designed to become as efficient as possible. This enabled us to conserve energy when we didn't know when our next meal would be. Now that most of our exercise comes from intentional workouts and not chasing down a buffalo or foraging for berries, we can easily fall into a rut of doing the same thing every time we throw on our workout clothes. After eight to twelve weeks,[4] though, your body adapts to this. Efficiency is great when planning a day full of errands or transporting multiple children to practices and games, all of which are obviously across town from each other. Not so much when you're looking for physical results.

Changing your workouts or even the type of weight you're using keeps efficiency at bay.

Mental excitement

Who doesn't love jumping into something new? I admit that while I try to maintain balance all year long, the scales literally and figuratively tip the other way by mid-December. As much as I try to attend Christmas parties and not eat too much, this is a true struggle for me. By month's end, I'm saturated. I'm tired of chocolate and wine and want an excuse to cancel all social events to eat my weight in green vegetables. My husband and I do this together. I flip through my favorite cookbooks and sites, looking for new healthy recipes to try. I establish a new workout routine. Dare I say it's exciting? The promise of sleeping well, feeling great, and working out in the mornings allures me. It's enough to keep me from quickly getting burned out.

After the "off-season" of the holidays, switching up my fitness keeps me excited. It gives me a new challenge. How much weight can I lift today? How far can I run? Can I get one more sprint in? All of these give me that push to lace up my shoes when I otherwise may not.

Since turning forty, I realized the best way to stay injury-free is by implementing periodization. Granted, it wasn't an intentional shift telling myself, "Amy, you are now going to apply periodization to your workouts." But I realized moving in different ways makes me feel best.

Not sure how to include periodization in your workouts? Consider incorporating the following into your workouts or routines.

Mobility

"If I could have done one thing differently when I was younger, it would be to do more mobility," said my friend who is about ten years older than I am. Mobility is a type of exercise that increases your range of motion and your control of the muscles that surround each joint. It's a sister to flexibility training and yoga. One main benefit of mobility is it intentionally takes your body in multiple directions. Our hip joint primarily moves forward and backward as we walk or sit. But if you look at the way God designed it, that femur (thigh bone) is intended and able to make a full circle within the ball-and-socket joint. Mobility training takes that femur and captures that ability. Same with the shoulder joint. Moving in different directions prevents overuse injury and keeps you fluid. Just be sure not to fetishize any of the movements you find you love.

Transverse exercises

Our body moves in three planes. Imagine a plate glass that can slice through your body. If you took the glass perpendicular to your body, dividing it into left and right halves, this is the sagittal plane. Dividing your body into a front and back is the frontal plane. The transverse plane bisects the body to create upper and lower halves. Any kind of twisting or rotating generally falls into a transverse plane.

Why do we care about transverse exercises? Because just like mobility, they encourage our body to move in multiple directions. This benefits both our muscles and fascia, which is the connective tissue covering our entire body. These exercises also train our bodies to move this way. Rarely does an injury from daily activity come in a perfect squat position. It's tripping on a dog bone and having to catch yourself from falling. It's reaching high for the paper towels, or even awkwardly carrying in the grocery bags we insist on getting in one trip. Life moves us in many directions; let's train our body to be ready for that.

Strength training modalities

Hopefully, you're convinced about the value of strength training after reading the chapter "I Don't Want to Bulk Up." If you have the means, consider using different sources of resistance: dumbbells, kettlebells, resistance bands, and your own body weight. If you really want to get technical, use one for three months, then switch to another.

Since hitting my forties, I've spent a lot of time trying to figure out the best way to exercise for this life stage. I can still execute heart-pumping, sweat-inducing workouts but not as often. I know the value of strength training. I now enjoy walking with friends more than running. And mobility workouts are now my secret sauce.

In other words, I enjoy a little bit of everything. If that sounds overwhelming, it's not meant to be. It's designed to give you the freedom to try whatever the heck you want. But one thing I do know: doing the same thing over and over will not be beneficial long-term. And there's certainly not one right way to exercise. Figure out what works for you, and embrace switching it up every now and then. You can even count weight if you want.

The Simple Take:
Try changing up your workout routine and how you
move every now and then to discover better results and
prevent injury.

30-Minute Mobility

If you've never tried mobility, here's your chance. Find the video link in your resource guide for a thirty-minute mobility workout with me. Or follow along below:

Set a timer and do each movement **45–60** seconds. Start with **45** seconds to allow yourself time to transition. After you've done the set a few times, increase to **60** seconds.

Cat cow

Hip circles

Individual hip circles

90/90s (internal and external rotation)

Reverse tabletop

Kneeling t-spine twist

Kneeling t-spine with lateral leg and reach, alternating sides

Wide low squat w/twist to bent-over hamstring stretch with hip shifts

Plank to pigeon, alternating sides (optional: add shoulder tap)

Wide squat with elbow to knee twist, alternating sides (roll wrists)

Plank to runners pose to twist, alternating sides

Down dog to under cross-leg, alternating sides

Kneeling hip flexor stretch 3 ways: raise arms up and down; across body; reach side to side

Bear to shooter slow

Supine knee twist

Boat to twist

Plank to knee to elbow

Folded cross-leg stretch

Quadruped diagonal stretch

Cat cow

Child's pose

CHAPTER NINETEEN

To lose weight, I need to exercise more and eat less

Some women swear they'd have twelve babies if they didn't have to deal with the toddler years and beyond. They love cuddling, nursing, and cooing their eight-pound blessings. They don't mind the crying or sleepless nights.

I am not one of these women. Newborns were hard. My actual newborns were not hard: none of my boys experienced colic, jaundice, or excessive gassiness. The newborn stage by itself was challenging for me. Like I've mentioned, I like rules. Brand-new humans do not follow rules, especially that of "sleep in the dark and be awake during the day." One of my sons used to take at least forty-five minutes to fall asleep every night. I tried nightly massages with lavender lotion. Bedtime nursing with instrumental music. Endless circles pacing our cul-de-sac.

Every time I figured out a way to get him to sleep well, that lasted a couple of weeks and something would change. His little body developed so quickly. What worked well tended to shift as fast as a toddler's demeanor when told "no." This frustrated me. I wanted to go back to what I knew worked before. But change is normal, and we can't always do what we've done. My son still takes a long time to fall asleep, even when he's exhausted. However, I'm pretty sure he would not want me to give him a lavender lotion massage. He loves me and I love him, but hairy man legs and mom massages are an awkward combination.

This is true in my health as well. When I want to lose a few pounds, I tend to go back to what I've always done and what has worked in the past.

My husband and I reserve January for strict eating, no wine, and little social engagement. It's such a blast. My husband executes January perfectly. His "on-or-off" philosophy serves him well as we buckle down. January is "on," while wine- and dessert-filled December is "off." Me? I do great. I cut out all my chocolate, increase the foods my body needs, and decrease the ones it doesn't. I am diligent, disciplined, and determined.

This lasts three days. Seventy-two hours, seventy-four if I'm lucky. And then I am mentally done. I'm tired of diligence, discipline, and determination. For many years, these three days were all my body needed to reset and get back to its set point in weight. I felt better, my body responded, and I was back to where my weight naturally wanted to be.

If that didn't work, I added something else in my back pocket. I just needed to increase my exercise duration and intensity. Simple as that, and in a few six-mile runs, indoor cycle classes, or two-a-day workouts, I'd be set. If I couldn't control my eating, then I could control my exercise, darn it!

This rhythm of exercise more, eat less lasted for most of my late twenties and thirties. Before that, I'm not sure. I don't think it ever occurred to me to restrict food in my early twenties. Did I start my junior year of college by swearing off sweets and Bud Light? Sadly, I think not.

In hindsight, it is not surprising I entered my forties with one injury or another. Overexercising from January through November for years caught up with me. My feet hurt all the time. My piriformis, a small muscle hidden beneath the gluteus maximus (your biggest butt cheek), complained. Twinges and tweaks told me they were tired of being so taxed.

If injuries were a wake-up call, my body was frequently setting the alarm clock at its loudest level. No sooner was one injury resolved than another one appeared. So, I started listening. Quite literally, actually. I found some podcasts that focused on fitness and aging. I began reading trade articles on how to train aging clients. As I learned more about my body and how her needs change over time, we developed a more respectful relationship.

I realized I had to take what I knew about eating less and exercising more and trash it. What worked before now will not. The same body that once thrived on long, intense sessions every day could no longer do so. Starving myself did more harm than good. Most of the rules recommending I exercise more and eat less come from studies focused on college-aged men,[1] not on women twice that age with different hormones. If I wanted to take care of my body, I needed to change my approach.

Exercising more and eating less is no longer my approach. I'd love it if you joined me in breaking this rule. I know I've talked a lot about finding contentment in our wonderfully made bodies, but I also realize sometimes we want to lose a few pounds to get to a weight we feel better in or that is healthier for us.

Here are six lessons I've learned about weight management since turning forty.

1. Long, intense sessions are not necessary

Hopefully, I've already convinced you that consistent one-hour sweat sessions are not what our body needs, so I won't rehash it completely here. If it's been a minute since you read Chapter 14, here's a recap:

- Something is better than nothing.
- Your favorite workout might better serve you shortened.
- Lose the two- to three-minute breaks during strength training workouts to shorten your time.
- Increase your metabolism through NEAT, not long exercise sessions.

2. My body needs to move in different ways

If you're lucky, you've found a way you love to move. Perhaps it's walking with friends, churning out rotations, cycling on a stationary bike, or flipping tires at a CrossFit gym. These tend to be our fallbacks when it's time to go back to what worked well. We know we met our goals before with these techniques; therefore, we believe if we just do them again, we will find success.

Perhaps. More than likely, though, if you continue to fall back to your tried-and-true ways, they will become tired and false. Why?

Your body thrives on efficiency.

We discussed this in the last chapter "There's One Right Way to Exercise." To recap, this is a lifesaving mechanism developed long before we had gym memberships and stability shoes. When our bodies didn't know when the next meal would come, they conserved as much energy as possible. They learned rhythms and habits and found the path of least resistance in making that happen. In short, our bodies became efficient at doing the same tasks.

Your body still does this. You may find yourself on the same bike every Monday, Wednesday, Friday, and Saturday for indoor cycling. At first, I bet you saw an increase in your endurance and lost some weight if that was part of your goal. Do this long enough, however, and you'll see fewer results. Your body starts to predict what you want it to do and becomes more efficient. Likewise, if the fifteen-pound weights that used to be challenging during a chest press no longer create soreness or increased strength, you've reached a strength plateau. Plateaus are what efficiencies love. After all, it's easier to navigate a flat terrain than a rocky mountain. When you began that chest press and could only complete eight repetitions, you found yourself sore and tender the next day. After a while, you easily completed fifteen. The space between the eight and fifteen created results because you were out of the efficiency zone.

When you change your workouts, that inefficiency (and sometimes awkwardness) has its benefits. Your metabolism increases as it has to work harder to perform the movements. If weight loss is a goal of yours, consider changing things up and seeing how your body responds.

You risk injury by going back to what has always worked.

Overtraining is the excessive frequency, volume, or intensity of training, resulting in fatigue (which is also caused by a lack of proper rest and recovery).[2] Fascia, the connective tissue that covers your body from head to toe, is designed to move multidirectionally. When it's not asked to move in different ways, it binds up. This causes it to pull and take the muscle with it. Sometimes a twinge in your knee is actually fascia pulling from the outer edge of your thigh. Additionally, unless the workout that has always worked includes a comprehensive program, chances are you're using one set of muscles significantly more than the other. Diving into the "exercise more, eat less" mindset often puts us into the default mode of what we know and love and forces our muscles to move in the same direction over and over and over.

3. Strength training is essential

We've already discussed the value of strength training and how it will not make you bulky. But for the purpose of this conversation, I want to revisit one of the benefits mentioned. Strength training increases your resting metabolic rate—your metabolism. If you've heard your metabolism slows down as you age, that's because we tend to lose muscle. This is called *sarcopenia*. It's a natural progression of our muscles, but we can slow that progression, and metabolism loss, by keeping strong muscles.

4. Rest matters, and it's hard to rest if I'm exercising more

Depending on your view of rest, I have good news or bad news. As we age, our body takes more time to put itself back together. Sleep is the number-one recovery tool, yet we sometimes neglect that in the name of productivity (I am guilty of this sometimes myself).

Rest allows your muscles to replenish and repair. After a tough workout, we've depleted the glycogen stores in our muscles that helped fuel said workout. Our body then takes the carbohydrates we consume and replenishes the muscles with glycogen, then takes the protein to repair the microtears we caused. Hitting the gym more often and with harder intensity doesn't allow the body to adequately go through this process. We will delve into rest thoroughly in the next chapter. Until then, know that rest days are critical.

5. My hormones have changed

As much as I'd like to get into the changes our body experiences hormonally and how this affects our workouts, that's beyond the scope of this book. However, I can provide the basic gist.

During the fertility years, our body's estrogen and progesterone levels are relatively high and consistent. Enter perimenopause, however, and the graph changes. Progesterone drops, and estrogen becomes confused. It's inconsistent at best, up during some times and down during others.

Besides managing our reproductive system, our hormones drive other aspects.

As Dr. Jade Teta explains in his Metabolic Renewal program, developed for women over forty, *"At certain times of the month when estrogen is a little bit higher, you can eat more, tolerate more stress, and your workouts will be intensified."*[3]

Progesterone helps stabilize mood, blocks the action of stress hormones like cortisol, and results in the body being less able to tolerate extreme diet and exercise approaches.[4]

Why does this matter? Because these hormones, along with others, affect your metabolism and workouts. They are complex hormones that impact our fat storage and burning capabilities. The food we eat and the way we move impact our hormones and vice versa. It's not all about calories in vs. calories out anymore. If you'd like more information on Dr. Teta's Metabolic Renewal program, visit his website: JadeTeta.com.

6. My body needs food in a different way now

I wish points one through five were enough to help me drop a few pounds when I want to. It's too bad this chapter doesn't end with, "Since instituting these steps, my body feels better, has fewer injuries, and I am able to move in all the ways I loved. I've continued eating in all the ways I loved as well. I lost weight when I needed to trim down by employing all these tactics."

As Lee Corso on ESPN's *College GameDay* likes to declare, "*Not so fast.*" Despite changing how I exercise and rest, a few metrics inched up, including that dreaded scale. It bothered me. I recognize this is counter to my message of appreciating and caring for our God-created bodies, no matter what they look like. Guilty as charged. But I also knew my body's set point and where it thrived.

I admit: My ego played a part as well. I'm a personal trainer, after all. While I pride myself on being "real-sized," I don't want to be dismissed because of my size.

I had a revelation: I'd spent a lot of time evaluating how best to move my body in my forties. Maybe it was time to reevaluate how I ate. Just like it was time to perform fewer high-intensity days and more transverse workouts, maybe it was time to eat differently. The challenge was figuring out how to do so within the self-imposed boundaries of treats and grace.

I needed to give my eating the same respect I'd given my exercise and consider doing something different.

Enter my friend Kandice, whom I'd been watching for about a year. She had begun a new lifestyle program that included workouts and nutrition. After several months, she told me how much better she felt and that she thought I'd love the program as well. When I asked her what it entailed, she told me whole-food nutrition (yes, I can get on board with that), intermittent fasting (but I love breakfast!), carb cycling (what the heck is that anyway?), and macro counting (no, thank you very much). I've tried tracking before and hated the obsession that went along with it.

The revelation ricocheted back: Yes, it's different than what I do and like. Maybe that's what I need. I swallowed a big piece of humble pie, called Kandice, and proceeded to interview her. Literally. I peppered her with questions and recorded it for my *Graced Health* podcast. (You can find this as a bonus episode to Season 1: "What is FASTer Way to Fat Loss? And all my other questions." I've also included a link in the online resource download.)

She explained the program in more detail and covered it all in grace and a healthy mindset. I decided to give it a shot. I made some changes. I paid more attention to my protein intake and realized I consumed more dietary fat than my body needed (even if it was healthy fat). Snacks not made in nature were dramatically reduced (though I still do love me some gluten-free pretzels every now and then). Against my desire, I tracked what I ate. Admittedly, I didn't love that part, but it helped me become aware of some eating patterns that needed tweaking. I didn't consume less food; I just consumed it differently with the right mix of carbs, fats, and proteins. I lengthened the amount of time between my last meal and first meal. I dropped the traditional breakfast time and instead ate my first meal around 11:00 a.m. Six weeks later, I still felt a little wobbly in everything, but I could tell this was the right step for me nutritionally. Six weeks after that, I found my rhythm and seemed to be on my way. My body responded, I found my set point again, and I felt more confident in my gym and street clothes.

It's been over a year now, and I still utilize many tenets of the program. I don't track my food as often, but have a better sense of how to balance out my day. I still wait until around 11:00 a.m. to eat, a type of intermittent fasting. My eating is a cross between the FASTer Way to Fat Loss program and intuitive eating. My daily choices are made from knowing what fuels my body best but not being overly focused on it. Granted, sometimes I take this freedom a little too far and find myself resetting for a few weeks.

I'm not convinced the program I used is the right one for everyone. Just because I found success with it doesn't mean it's right for you. But changing how I ate and not how little I ate was key.

I'm not the same person as age-thirty Amy. Among other things, I'd like to think I'm less judgy and more empathetic. My understanding and stance on social and racial issues have changed right along with my aging body.

My body is different as well. It used to be that to lose weight, I simply needed to exercise more and eat less. That doesn't work anymore. But even though that was a simple process, I appreciate the new one now. I have more time with shorter workouts, I don't get bored doing the same thing over and over, and best of all, I now know little things about my body that help it run well.

The Simple Take:
As you age, eating less and exercising more may not be
the best way for you to lose weight. You may need to
change how you eat but not how much you eat.

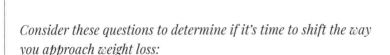

Consider these questions to determine if it's time to shift the way you approach weight loss:

1. What are your go-to methods when you try to lose weight?

2. Do any of them still work?

3. What may be an alternative approach?

4. Is there a science-based program you've been interested in trying but haven't?

If you answer any of the following questions with a yes, it may be time to change your approach if your goal is to lose weight:

1. Do you regularly exercise more than an hour?

2. Have you been doing the same movement for more than six months?

3. Do you incorporate strength training into your movement?

4. Do you forgo rest days in the name of losing weight?

5. Are you over the age of forty?

6. Do you severely restrict your caloric intake?

CHAPTER TWENTY

No rest for the weary

In college, I was an okay student. I earned decent grades, but "earn" is the operative word. Every "A" on that report card came from hours of studying. One Sunday during my sophomore year, I sat on my bed studying for Tuesday's Business Calculus test. I struggled in that class and desperately needed a good grade. The Oklahoma April weather allowed me to open the window and get some fresh air as I worked. Outside I heard the intermittent cheers of an entire city. Our basketball team was fighting for a slot in the NCAA tournament's Final Four. We hadn't reached the Elite Eight in thirty years, and this year looked promising. It's still one of my biggest collegiate regrets that I ignored the game and studied for a test I didn't even make an A on.

Each semester I crammed for finals, sacrificing sleep for a twenty-four-hour, color-coded schedule (I don't recommend this). And with each final test, I immediately packed my car, drove an hour-and-a-half home, and crashed. My brain was toast, and the thirteen hours of sleep several days in a row proved it. My body and brain needed rest.

In fitness, rest days are imperative. Yet scroll through Pinterest, and you'll see shaming for wanting to take a day off:

- There's plenty of time to rest when you're done.
- No rest for the best.
- Ambition has no rest.
- No sleep, no rest until you're the best.
- No days off.

And the one that really makes my skin crawl:

- Rest day? That's why no one will remember your name.

These mantras are absurd. I hope this chapter helps you see why.

Physical rest days are essential

Whether you're running, strength training, high-intensity interval training, or engaging in any activity that is strenuous and may leave you sore, you need a rest day. This is due to microtears your muscles develop when put under stress. They need time to replenish and repair. Specifically, rest allows time for the fibroblasts to repair muscle tissue.[1] Fibroblasts are a type of cell that help promote wound healing (and those microtears in your muscles are wounds).

A rest day also allows your blood to deliver oxygen and nutrients to those taxed cells. If you're constantly placing your muscles and systems under exercise stress, they can't receive the elements needed for their repair.[2]

Muscles constantly under stress do not thrive. At a minimum, they won't perform well. When taxed beyond their ability to recover, they act out in the form of overtraining syndrome. This results in muscle strains, stress fractures, and joint pain. Then guess what? You get too many rest days because you can't do what you want to do.

How long should you rest your muscles? The general consensus among fitness professionals is to allow forty-eight hours in between working the same muscle groups. For example, if you focus on strength training your shoulders, biceps, and triceps on Monday, you should avoid taxing these muscles again until Wednesday. Tuesday's workout can be used for something else, like a leg-day focus, walk, or high-intensity interval.

I hear a lot of confusion about rest days. I understand. For example, can I run after a leg day? What about a bodyweight-based class after an upper-body day? Yes to both of these, by the way. The key is establishing how intensely your muscles were strained. Strength training can, and should, stress your muscles to the point of microtears. This is what causes stronger muscles. Those microtears are repaired and rebuilt, causing thicker and bigger muscles. Soreness represents those small tears (and your hard work, as we discussed).

Here's a general litmus test: if you're sore, you need a rest day or need to take down the intensity to a low or moderate level. Give those muscles forty-eight hours to repair and replenish. You can do something else in the meantime by focusing on a different body part or by lowering your intensity. Walking or even endurance running after a leg day is fine because the intensity is lower. You don't break down those muscles while walking. Rest days also help bring those nutrients and fibroblasts to your muscles to aid in repair. If you're super sore, gently moving may be just what you need.

How to approach a rest day

Rest days in the fitness world have a million different definitions. Whatever the definition, we need them. Regardless of your fitness level, you still need to provide your body with that day or two of replenishment and restoration. You don't earn a rest day once you get to a certain ability or size. My rest day typically means I only walk my dog, Grace, or I'm gently moving through mobility movements. My friend Kandice from the last chapter may not exercise on her rest days but is intentional about getting 10,000 steps in. As a goat farmer, this comes a little more naturally, but she's still aware of her movement.

Here are some ways you can utilize your day off to repair and replenish your body and soul:

- Prayer walk (Casually walk down your street or neighborhood, specifically praying for each family.)
- Yoga
- Gentle self-myofascial release using a foam roller or a massage stick (May especially be helpful if you're sore![3] Remember I've provided a quick demo video in "No Pain, No Gain.")

- Bike ride (Think parade pace, not race pace.)
- Nap
- Mobility ("There's One Right Way to Exercise" includes a mobility workout and an accompanying video.)
- Stretch
- Playtime with your kids in their chosen activity

What about a couch-based Netflix binge? It's not preferred, but if that is what gives you the energy to get back at it, then go for it. After all, we aren't here to blindly follow the rules. We are here to figure out what is best for us.

Mental rest days are important as well

Let's be honest: Figuring out how and when to move, what to eat, and how to successfully execute all this amidst an already full day is exhausting. Physically, yes, but mentally as well. At times, I just need a mental break from trying to figure it all out. Taking a day off is not a failure. It's allowing your body and brain to rest so you can begin the next day with more excitement. Even as a lifelong fitness enthusiast, I feel a little mentally lighter on the days I previously scheduled rest. As a bonus, I have more time in my day to check off that to-do list, which pleases my goal-setting heart. Maybe, just maybe, I'll get a little self-care in as well.

Even God took a rest day

After God took six days to create light, water, sky, land, planets, stars, creatures, and man, He took a rest day. Literally.

> *By the seventh day God had finished the work he had been doing; so on the seventh day he rested from all his work. Then God blessed the seventh day and made it holy, because on it he rested from all the work of creating that he had done.*

Genesis 2:2–3

Not only did God rest, He deemed it holy. Later, He asked the Isra-elites to trust Him and take a rest day. Every morning, He provided food in the form of manna, but He instructed them to take the sev-enth day as Sabbath and not gather food (Ex. 16:26). When they went out anyway, they found nothing and had to rely on the extra portion they were instructed to gather the day before.

Four commandments into the famous Ten, we read God's instruc-tions to remember the Sabbath day:

> *Six days you shall labor and do all your work, but the seventh day is a sabbath to the Lord your God. On it you shall not do any work, neither you, nor your son or daughter, nor your male or female servant, not your animals, nor any foreigner residing in your towns.*
>
> Exodus 20:9

Jesus rested too. In Mark 6:31, Jesus said to His disciples, "*Come away by yourselves to a secluded place and rest a while.*" After teaching on the Sermon on the Mount (which no doubt felt like a marathon), Jesus retreated with His disciples to a boat. I'm sure they all needed to get away. Jesus laid down with His pillow to rest and slept through a storm. When the panicked disciples woke Him, two words calmed the storm: *Be still.* While the primary message of this story is prob-ably to learn to trust Christ in the storm, could it also be that we see His physical and mental need to rest? And maybe we just need to be still sometimes?

I know God didn't specifically mention exercise here, but I think we get the gist. No matter what we are doing, it's important to take a break. A Sabbath day allows us to replenish our relationship with Christ; a physical rest day allows us to replenish and repair our body. It's hard and humbling to put down our never-ending to-do list, but it also honors the fact that God is God and we are not. If He takes a rest day, so should we.

It's worth mentioning one of the most impactful books on rest I've read: *Sacred Rest* by Dr. Saundra Dalton-Smith. If your body feels fine but something else just doesn't feel right, I recommend checking out her book to see what kind of rest you need and how to obtain it. Her insight into the many ways we replenish ourselves is revealing.

Unexpected rest days happen

But what if something happens to my day and my planned workout just doesn't get done? This happens too. Pre-kids, my days used to be predictable and easily manipulated. If work ran late, I simply attended a later class at the YMCA. Or I went home and ran. My husband was the only person I was accountable to, and he understood my need to work out as he needed it too. Add babies and kids to the mix, however, and workout schedules got more complicated. It started with sleepless nights with a sick baby, then ever-changing nap times. School brought organized activities, practices, and early-morning Saturday games.

Life happens. While I'm an advocate for regular workouts, I'm not an advocate for feeling shame when they don't happen as scheduled. Missing a workout does not mean you aren't going to meet your goals. It doesn't mean you've failed the plan, whatever plan that is. It simply means you didn't get your workout in for the day. Give yourself some grace, and get back into it the next day.

My aging body is a little more vocal about her need for rest days. She used to quietly obey my command to keep going or add another workout. But just like I'm more attuned to my mental health and emotions now than ten years ago, my body speaks up more now as well. She sets boundaries. She demands time off. I'm learning to comply. When we cooperate, we are more successful. I give her rest, and she responds by allowing me to run fast or lift heavy.

If I may, I'd like to reframe some of those Pinterest memes I mentioned earlier to help us not only embrace but also welcome rest days:

- Rest when you need it.
- The best rest.
- Ambition includes rest.
- Sleep and rest make you the best.
- Take a day off.

And a new rule to live by:

- No rest leads to weariness.

Rest days do not mean failure. They are an active path to progress in disguise.

The Simple Take:
Rest days allow for your muscles to replenish and rejuvenate. Sometimes they are planned; other times they are thrown at us. Regardless, allowing one or two rest days a week will help you achieve your fitness goals and prevent injury.

How can you appreciate your own rest days? Take a few minutes and jot down three ways you can spend a rest day. If there's no movement, that's okay. Permission granted to write down shows or books you want to read in your time off!

1. _____

_____

_____

_____

2. _____

_____

_____

_____

3. _____

_____

_____

_____

PART THREE: COOL DOWN

We warmed up by exploring our body image and the foundations of why we take care of our bodies. Then we did our own exercise of discussing nourishment, nutrients, and movement.

We now enter our cooldown phase. In our workouts, this is the time to put our bodies back together. In this book, it's the time to wrap everything up. I hope this cooldown is enough for you to consider all we've discussed, shaken up, and helps you put your thoughts surrounding your body and health back together.

CHAPTER TWENTY-ONE

It's a waste of time if I don't lose weight

*M*y friend sent me a text that voiced the frustrations of so many I've heard over the years. She'd been working on her health for a few months, getting up early to work out and changing her eating habits. After six weeks, her scale showed no affirmation of the hard work she'd been doing. In other words, she hadn't lost any weight. You can imagine her frustration.

She wrote, "I'm working my literal butt off, and my head is beginning to tell my heart this isn't working because it's taking forever." She expressed dismay with the program she was on in that it was too strict and time-consuming to prep. On top of that, she felt like she received different nutritional guidance with different programs she looked into: "There is so much information out there, and it all discounts the other. How do I do this without wasting any more time?"

Can we just stop for a minute for a show of hands? Who has felt this pain? I have. And if you're like the many, many women I've had conversations with, you may have too. My friend captured so many points in one text.

We already discussed the nutritional aspect of this. I hope I've convinced you to figure out what works best for you in "There's One Best Diet." Let's delve into the second part of her text: "How do I do this without wasting any more time?" In other words, how can we stay motivated?

Remember—or identify—your why

If you've gotten this far, may I assume you're interested in living a healthy lifestyle? May I ask why you want to do this? This is your "why." It shouldn't be because I, or any other person or program, give you ways...rules...of doing it. Your favorite celebrity, health coach, or podcaster does not have that authority over you. Your own unique reason for focusing on your health is what will keep you motivated through those moments of frustration.

Your why does not have to be complicated. Having something simple to cling to when everything else feels slippery may be exactly what you need. I polled my Facebook friends as to what drove them. Many of them said something along the lines of "When I take care of myself, I feel better physically and emotionally." Others wanted to set a good example for their children or were trying to change the course of their health after watching their parents suffer. I've spoken with a handful of people who had children later in life and want to be around as long as possible. Here's one of my favorite Facebook responses: "To feel good. Wellness takes work!" Yes, it does. But when we put in the work, we can and do feel better.

Recognize the effect on your sphere of influence

I have a new client whose goals echo so many others. As a woman in her late thirties, she's invested plenty of time into her job, children, and husband and just wants to take care of herself. We train over Zoom twice a week. One of her daughters frequently joins us. This four-year-old adorably mimics her mom. The other one may not plank with us, but she sees her mom making positive changes. My client told me her daughter also likes to pretend that she runs a workout and tells her sister how to exercise. Without realizing it, my client not only invested in taking care of herself but also in teaching her daughters to do so as well.

Your people see you. Your coworkers hear your tales of getting up early. Your children see your sweaty gym clothes. Your spouse notices the healthier options at dinner (I hope without complaints). Your hard work influences more people than you know. We don't do this for other people, but it doesn't hurt when others are influenced by what we're doing.

Assess how you feel

Pay attention to how your body responds to your efforts. Sometimes even the smallest wins are enough to keep us moving. You may notice other ways your body is responding to your effort. Consider these.

Functionality

Some of the most successful wins that my clients have experienced are not huge changes in the scale or even in measurements. They've experienced wins like getting out of bed without groaning and maintaining stamina on a European tour that was heavy on the walking. One client shared a story of being sideswiped by her energetic dog and popping back up after landing on the ground rather than nursing a broken ankle.

Body aches

Moving your body and eating well reduces the levels of inflammation in your body. Inflammation is what often causes general bodily discomfort. When I overindulge in jelly beans, my left hip wakes me up at night throbbing. When you put mostly God-given vegetables, fruits, plants, and lean meats in your body, you may find you are less inflamed.

Waste

I'm the official potty-humor instigator in my house. To the eye rolls of my people, I'll address this important question: How is your poop? When you're hydrated and eating plenty of fiber, your bathroom time should be relatively quick and without issue. Multiple and difficult plop, plop, plops may indicate you're dehydrated or haven't had enough fiber. Or, if you poop like a goose, you may be eating something that doesn't agree with you. If your bathroom time is improving, your time spent drinking your water and eating your vegetables is certainly not wasted.

Fitness performance

Continuing to show up will result in better performance. Whether you see an increase in your endurance or the weight you are lifting, over the course of time you'll see results. Notice the small rewards.

Energy levels

Energy is a fairly subjective thing to track. But most of us can recognize when we have more of it. And I can tell you that when I'm crawling into bed to close my eyes for thirty minutes each day, it's probably related to my nutrition. By the same token, if I take several days off from formal exercise, I find myself sluggish. Even some of the teens I've spoken with can make this association. Talk about the opposite of wasting time...eliminating even a thirty-minute nap helps me check off more of my to-do list.

Increased immunity

A poor diet and lack of physical activity are associated with negative health consequences. Regular moderate activity is beneficial for boosting your immune system, particularly upper respiratory tract infections. Eating a wide variety of fruits and vegetables may do the same.[1] If you make it through the winter with nary a cold, give yourself a pat on the back for eating the foods that protect and fuel you well.

Slowing cognitive decline

Many of us have watched a loved one suffer through the monster of dementia or Alzheimer's disease. Dr. Sanjay Gupta shares several pieces of research in his book *Keep Sharp* that connect exercise to enhanced brain function and resiliency to disease. In fact, he promotes exercise as the single most important thing in slowing cognitive decline. I realize this may not be something you can recognize in the moment, but knowing that exercise affects the later part of your life may help keep you motivated.

Emotional and mental state

Those endorphins mentioned in "Walking Isn't a Real Workout" are legit. Despite the frustration, how's your emotional health? Are you more resilient with the ups and downs of the day? Perhaps you're able to communicate your emotions better or are allowing yourself to actually feel all the feels rather than numb them with food, alcohol, or endless scrolling.

My dog, Grace, tends to get antsy if she goes more than a couple of days without a walk. She's unsettled and frenetic. She barks at falling leaves or squirrels frolicking in the yard. Honestly, it's somewhat annoying. I realized this morning I hadn't taken her out in a few days, and her mental and physical state missed it. While I didn't have a lot of time, I put a leash on her. After just one mile, she was back to her normal self. Currently, she's settled and snoozing comfortably by my feet. My head gets this way as well. Exercise breaks through cobwebs. I focus better and snap at my people less. I'm also less annoying when I regularly exercise.

As researcher Kelly McGonigal, PhD, writes in her book *The Joy of Movement*:

> *In humans, exercising three times a week for six weeks increases neural connections among areas of the brain that calm anxiety. Regular physical activity also modifies the default state of the nervous system so that it becomes more balanced and less prone to fight, flight, or fright.* [2]

By the way, if you're struggling to find ways your body feels better, be like Dory from *Finding Nemo* and just keep swimming. Your initial response to a new form of exercise may not be how you feel after you do it repeatedly. [3] Just like coffee was an acquired taste for me, enjoyment of movement may take a bit.

Use the scale as one tool but not the only tool

Even after all these words I've written, I still pull out my scale from time to time. However, my relationship with it has changed over the years. I consider one of my greatest victories to have stepped on it recently, looked down to see that number several pounds heavier than I expected, cocked my head to the side, and proclaimed, "Huh. That's interesting." But it took many years and tears to get there.

Merriam-Webster.com defines weight as "the force with which a body is attracted toward the earth or a celestial body by gravitation and which is equal to the product of the mass and the local gravitational acceleration."[4] Your weight doesn't define progress or your worth as a human.

The scale fluctuates. Yes, you may have muscle or adipose changes. It also may reflect a salty or high-carb meal, monthly cycle variations, alcohol intake, or even overexercising (your muscles will retain water after several hard workouts in a row).

As I told my friend, don't worry about the scale. If your waist or hips or thighs or big toe are losing circumference, you are finding success. My friend actually had lost inches; the scale didn't reflect that because her body had grown muscle and lost fat. Muscle tissue is more dense than fat and thus takes up less space.

Contrary to public opinion, muscle doesn't weigh more than fat. A pound is a pound is a pound. But the space they take up differ. Visualize a gallon-sized bag of cotton candy at your local ballpark. At 220 calories, this kid-favorite treat is pure sugar and food coloring. Four calories is equivalent to one gram, so that's fifty-five grams of sugar. One teaspoon of sugar is also four grams, so if we divide fifty-five by four, we are holding a little less than fourteen teaspoons of sugar in that fluffy bag. Now take that same bag and instead of cotton candy put fourteen sugar cubes in it. Those sugar cubes worth one teaspoon take up less space even though the caloric count is the same.

Likewise, a pound of muscle takes up less space than a pound of adipose.

Yes, I just used a cotton candy and sugar example to explain the difference in space that muscle and fat consume. I realize the irony here. But when you begin to develop more muscle tissue and lose adipose, your body shows the difference even if the scale doesn't.

Remember, any effort you put into your health is not wasted time, even if life throws a curveball

One of my childhood friends experienced the trauma of divorce. Her parents were heavily involved in their church, and the dissolution of their marriage was shocking. In my naive fourteen-year-old view on Christian living, I commented once that I thought bad things didn't happen to Christians. The incredulous look I received back didn't need her response: "Oh yes. Bad things happen to Christians. All the time."

Unfortunately, this is also true in our health. I can't responsibly leave you without one gentle reminder: Taking care of yourself is not a magical bubble of protection. Bad things also happen to healthy people. Yes, we have research touting the benefits of exercise and eating well. It's all true. But it's not a guarantee. On a small scale, I've seen this in my hypertension battle. I've also seen it in friends who finish half marathons and then get diagnosed with breast cancer. All the kale, quinoa, and mobility workouts in the world don't prevent heartache. We lose jobs, children, parents. We receive unexpected and unwelcome diagnoses. We find ourselves in a global pandemic.

If I've learned one thing from *Everything Happens* with Kate Bowler, one of my favorite podcasts, it's not to prescribe anything during times of heartache and loss. So I won't. No magical green smoothies. No promising supplements. No healing diet.

Everything does happen. And if these things have happened to you, I'm sorry. I'm so, so sorry.

I wish I could provide a five-step process to heal through food and movement. I can't. But I can say these can still help your healing journey. On my podcast, I interviewed a physician's assistant with a world-renowned cancer treatment center. She shared how those entering treatment for cancer fare better when they have healthy nutritional and movement habits. Their bodies are better able to withstand the demands of treatment and the horrible side effects that come with it. Putting God-given foods in our body can help it function better, even when we can barely function. Being physically fit enables her patients to endure grueling treatment. Don't get me wrong: if chemotherapy leaves you only wanting to eat butter crackers, then eat them. If you're deep in grief and you can't get out of bed, stay in bed. Take the time you need to heal in whatever that way is.

Whatever your "thing" is, I want you to be able to deal with it without the shame of feeling like you caused it. You didn't. And wherever you are now, you can take whatever small step makes sense to you now. That may be a five-minute walk down the street and back, grabbing one extra vegetable with your lunch, or actually stopping with one piece of chocolate rather than one piece of six different types of chocolate (or maybe that's just me).

The steps you're taking are worth it. No healthy step is wasted effort, even if that journey was not one you signed up for.

You may not see the kind of results you want in the time you expect, but it's all worth it. I promise. Pay attention to the small ways your body and brain respond to your kindness. Because let's be clear: Taking care of your body is being kind to yourself.

The Simple Take:
The time you invest into taking care of yourself is
worth it, even if you don't achieve the kind of
results you are hoping for.

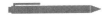

If you are questioning if it's all worth it, take inventory of these metrics. If possible, compare them to the beginning of your journey.

Assess where you are on a scale of 1-10 (10 is ideal), and compare that to your starting point.

- Functionality
- Body aches
- Waste
- Fitness performance
- Energy levels
- Immunity
- Emotional and mental state

CHAPTER TWENTY-TWO

Go hard or go home (Conclusion)

This book is my COVID-19 baby. In March 2020, when the world came to a screeching halt, I was inspired by a mentor who declared, "This time is for everyone who's ever said they want to write a book."

This mentor has since revised that statement. As quarantine life unfolded, it brought the loss of life and jobs, mental health issues, and overall discord and collective trauma. Managing work, online schooling, and a general shift in pretty much everything does not make for a good creative writing space. I believe we will see research and studies for years to come revealing long-term effects of those who tested positive and recovered, academic gaps, and how this impacted our mental health.

I'm grateful our family didn't experience any of this in 2020. Yes, we had to figure out new patterns and workspaces, but in general, we were spared from the traumatic effects.

Back to March 2020. Through my mentor's words and a consistent prompting by the Holy Spirit, I felt God calling me to focus more heavily on writing this book. So I did. But I didn't sit down and bang out all 60k+ words in a matter of days or weeks. Instead, I approached this goal with bite-size chunks of time to write five hundred words in random spaces of thirty minutes, following my heart for the day.

With such a sporadic writing schedule, one could say I didn't exactly give it my full effort.

I'd argue I did. It may look different than my colleague who wrote a full manuscript in three weeks, but I found the rhythm and pace that worked for me and my situation.

Did I *go hard* writing the message? Not really. But I got enough done, little by little, in a way that worked for me. Except for the one weekend I booked myself a little cabin in the woods (a glorious act of self-care), most of these words came in between endless meal prepping and lingering in the kitchen (disguised as cleaning) while my kids shared slivers of their heart.

It's a fitting analogy to our fitness and overall health.

The saying "Go hard or go home" is meant to encourage those exercising to give it their all or don't even bother...stay at home. We've been together long enough that you can probably surmise my feeling on this statement.

You actually don't have to give it your all every time you approach a workout. Remember Enough from "No Pain, No Gain?" She is the antithesis of "Go Hard or Go Home." She's also a lot more fun to hang out with. We've discussed the importance of rest and how gentle mobility workouts can promote an increased range of motion, stabilize joints, and prevent injury.

Part of my journey includes finding balance in my movement and food. I'm not always great about perfectly executing it, but I'm getting better. I hope and pray the words here help you find your own balance. The problem with balance, though, is it's not very exciting.

I've never seen a morning-show segment or BuzzFeed story about a mom who got up to walk a few miles most days (but hit snooze others); prepared lunch for her children (but sometimes let them buy lunch at school); tried to volunteer at their school (when it didn't conflict with work or other obligations); and provided dinner (as a mix of takeout, healthy meals, and fridge clean out). At the end of the day, though, she was content. She didn't go crazy in anything but she got the job done, whatever it was. She may have achieved balance in her day, but it's wasn't very sexy. Quite frankly, it doesn't make for a compelling story.

Isn't that what we all want, though? To be able to complete all our necessary tasks so nothing suffers? And going back to the beginning of our time together, isn't contentment something we need?

As for balance, what exactly is that? We hear of work/life balance. Balanced exercise. Balanced nutrition. Balanced government (hey, we can all dream).

Balanced health looks different for different people and in different seasons of life. For some, this means taking a thirty-minute walk after dinner. For others, it's rising before the sun and her people to complete a six-mile run or head to a barre class. Balanced health for new moms may simply be having enough time to shower, brush their teeth, and eat something while nursing the baby. The thought of sixty minutes of exercise sounds simultaneously heavenly and ridiculously elusive.

It wasn't until my forties that I started paying any attention to balanced health. As we've discussed, my previous seasons were extreme and ill-focused. Upon entering my forties, God taught me that in taking care of my body, I needed to set it up for long-term vibrancy. Every time I've trained for long-distance races (half marathons), my body acted out. One time my feet were in so much pain I had to wear stabilizing shoes all the time, including waterproof flip-flops while showering. Another left me with hip bursitis so bad I couldn't sit cross-legged for longer than about twelve and a half seconds.

These were not examples of vibrancy. I understand they are often side effects of ramping up for an event, whatever that may be. I began to wonder, though, if what I was doing to my body now would prevent me from doing what I wanted to do *later*.

Later, I want to sit on the floor with my grandchildren and play with the Thomas the Train tracks I've saved.

Later, I want to travel the world with my husband. I want to visit ancient ruins and historical places that require us to hike and climb.

Later, I want to get off the floor with ease.

If I live a fitness life in extremes, I may be decreasing my chances of vibrancy later. As a doctor once told my husband, "The strongest muscles in the world won't help if you can't bend down and pick up your car keys when they fall." I do want strong muscles. But I also want to be able to pop up and down off the floor and respond to life as it comes. These days, I'm caring less about how I look (though let's be honest, yes I do care) and more about how I function.

For me, balance now is the key to that.

It's not very sexy though. A great story does not come from doing a lot of different exercises so as not to burn one body part out. Telling someone I do a couple of days of strength training, a little running, a lot of walking, and mobility doesn't capture much attention. It certainly isn't very inspiring.

As my years progress, I hear people say, "I really don't care what I look like; I just want to be strong and healthy." I love this approach. Yes! We should all have this attitude.

I ask, though, Where's the model for this? Where is the example you can follow and think, "I can do that!"

My hope is you now have the model. You have permission to do what is best for you...not what the morning shows tout, the internet declares as the latest-and-greatest eating or exercise plan, or your favorite Instagram influencer does. Doing what is best for you may look completely different than what you've learned or expected, and that's okay. Play around with what you've learned here in order to figure it out.

We've covered quite a bit—from faith to food to fitness. I hope you downloaded all the resources and goodies that accompanied this book. After all, if I'm going to tell you to stop something, I want to give you an alternative to start.

My goal in this time together was to simplify things for you to take away any shame of feeling like your eating, movement, and/or body don't measure up. As I say in my podcast episodes, I leave you with this: What's the one simple take I hope you remember from reading this book? Your eating, movement, and body don't have to be perfect. You just need to move your body in a way that works for you and fuel it with God's foods so you can do what you are called to do. You are worth it.

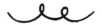

CONNECT WITH AMY

Connect with Amy

I invite you to stay in touch through my monthly journals at GracedHealth.com/monthly-updates. This is a fun, subscriber-only space that feels safe enough for me to be as snarky as I want while providing foods, recipes, movements, music, and other gems I think you'll enjoy. You can also find plenty of resources on the "Resources" tab over at GracedHealth.com. Whether you're looking for support in your food, fitness, or faith, I have you covered.

My *Graced Health* podcast episodes offer a mix of exercise science, faith-focused health, nutrition, and mental health. Depending on the conversation, we can cover a lot of ground. When I'm on the receiving end of episodes that provide a buffet's worth of data and information, I tend to choose one thing to walk away with. I need to simplify it. That's why at the end of most episodes I offer one simple thing to remember (and why I did the same for you in each chapter here).

In the spirit of simplicity, if you want to choose one way to stay connected, sign up for the monthly journals.

Finally, if this book blessed you, may I ask one thing? Please leave an honest review on Amazon, or share this book with a friend who could use some grace and balance.

ACKNOWLEDGMENTS

I always enjoy reading the acknowledgments at the end of the book. One statement I've seen mentioned multiple times is something to the effect of "it takes a lot of people to put a book together." *Your Worthy Body* is no exception. My name may be on the cover, but without the investment of others, I could not have developed this into something you are holding in your hands.

To my editors.

Andrea Barilla Editing and Writing Services, you provided the vision that I didn't know I needed. The reworks we wrestled through may have been harder than actually writing the first draft, but they made it infinitely better. As you promised, it was worth the time. Thanks for hearing me out in those challenging chapters and helping to formulate a clear structure.

Samantha Hanni, thank you for your dual role of editor and therapist. Your technical expertise is appreciated but so is your encouragement that I don't have to please everyone and that I don't have to apologize for so much. I'm sorry you had to tell me that so many times. Also, thank you for letting me use ALL CAPS (and sometimes parentheses) against your professional guidance.

To the creatives.

Rebecca Sutton, you took my words and gave them life as the interior designer. I never anticipated being so excited about how this booked looked on the inside.

Steve Kuhn, the cover of this book still takes my breath away. Well done. Thank you for listening to my fuzzy vision and then providing a clear product that offers peace, simplicity, and beauty.

Erin Bartels, thanks for seeing the forest when all I could see were the trees. You helped clarify the message of this entire book into 250 words for the back of the book and other marketing materials.

Lis Purdy, your eye behind the camera has always astounded me. Thank you for capturing my multifaceted personality in a still shot. And while your photography art is beautiful, your heart is even more so. Thank you for your friendship.

To my unknowing mentors.

Pete McCall, I'm pretty sure you're quoted more than any other person in this book, and with good reason. Thank you for educating enthusiasts and fitness professionals alike. I've learned so much from you, your articles, your *All About Fitness* podcast, and your books *Smarter Workouts* and *Ageless Intensity*.

Kathi Lipp, your faithful servitude to communicators is evidenced through the completion of this book. Because of your Communicator Academy, *Writing at the Red House* podcast, blog posts, speaker conference, and online lessons and challenges, I gained enough wisdom and confidence to take the next step and know it doesn't have to be perfect.

Chad R. Allen, I can only imagine the faith it took to leave professional publishing to help writers like myself get their books into the world. Thank you for your infinite wisdom through BookCamp and enduring countless questions about self-publishing vs. traditional publishing.

To my consultants.

As I mentioned, while I sometimes act like a know-it-all, I do not know it all. I'm grateful for the wisdom and guidance of those who helped confirm or clarify content related to their expertise: Emily Baker, Pastor Nathan Bryant, Pete McCall, and Rev. Donna Owusu-Ansah. Thank you all.

To the book team.

Betsy, Kristine, Kay, and Leslie, thank you for being early readers and providing feedback. Your honesty is valued. You told me what was confusing, how you felt, and what would make the message stronger. You also gave me the confidence to release chapter after chapter and to believe that the words were worth continuing to write.

Alison, Kristen, Sitel, Doris, Jennifer H., Jennifer K., and Lynn, thank you for trying the recipes in your own home, time, and budget. I never knew if they were actually going to work. I'm grateful you discovered the missing steps and ingredients. You also confirmed that I'm not the detail-oriented person I wish I was.

Kristine, your research was invaluable. I knew you were just the person with the right expertise and right heart to help me out. Thank you.

To a few other friends.

Kristen, in our early-morning training sessions, you allowed me to experiment with the movements that ended up as resources. Your patience with random "hey can I bounce something off you?" texts is also noted and appreciated.

Barbara, I'm not sure if you remember sitting in the car one day telling me I had a good writing voice. You said if I was ever interested in starting a blog you'd help me through the process. You did. And those words gave me the confidence to start. Thank you for planting that seed and for being the kind of friend everyone needs. And thank you, as well, for letting me experiment exercises and movements with you and Kristen.

Camisha, I believe our friendship is God-ordained. Chapter 4 is OUR chapter; you had just as much of a hand in it as I did. Thank you for patiently educating me about your perspective as a Black woman and walking with me through the chapter (figuratively and literally). The time spent on our neighborhood's sidewalks during the first Black Girls RUN! eRace Racism challenge are deeply cherished.

Laura, our early-morning walks are critical to my mental, spiritual and physical health. Thank you for your true interest in how this process was going and allowing me to often dominate at least two-and-a-half miles of our three miles (and some change) together.

And thank you to the countless others who have encouraged, supported, and inquired about this process. If you're wondering if I mean you, I do.

To my clients, past and present.

Thank you for trusting me with your bodies. We met and connected in various ways and you have your own goals, but I'm honored to be a part of your health journey. I do not take that lightly.

Debbie, you were my first personal training client. We met as you were putting yourself back together after a challenging season, and I'm genuinely honored to have been a part of that process.

To my parents.

Mom and Dad, my first memory of making a healthier food choice was switching from white Wonder to wheat bread. Talk about a sphere of influence (as discussed in Chapter 21). I witnessed you exercising in your own way and choosing nutritious foods. And of course, you provided a lot of nourishment along the way. Thank you and I love you. Sounds simple but is as genuine as it comes.

To my three men.

Being the husband and children of a health geek isn't easy. You hear way more about the fascia than you want and I know I'm bossy in the gym. Boys, I still tell you to eat your vegetables even though you're a foot taller than me. I'm working on all of this. Your love and support through the writing of this book cannot be described. You are my rock and keep me grounded. And one of you isn't afraid to say, "Come on Mom, you're better than that" when I have my own moments of insecurity or self-doubt. Thank you for letting me share snippets of our lives together even though two of you prefer to be off-the-grid. I love you all more than I can express.

To my friend, Jesus.

Without your grace and unselfish love I couldn't give grace and love to myself.

SOURCES

Introduction

1. Alyssa Roat, "What Does Agape Love Really Mean in the Bible?" Christianity.com, originally published December 20, 2019, https://www.christianity.com/wiki/christian-terms/what-does-agape-love-really-mean-in-the-bible.html.

2. Brené Brown, "Shame v. Guilt," *Brené Brown*, January 14, 2013, https://brenebrown.com/blog/2013/01/14/shame-v-guilt/#close-popup.

Chapter 1: I'm Supposed to Look a Certain Way

1. "Marilyn Monroe's True Size," The Marilyn Monroe Collection, accessed September 1, 2020, https://themarilynmonroecollection.com/marilyn-monroe-true-size/.

2. Vanessa Van Edwards, "Beauty Standards: See How Body Types Change Through History," Science of People, accessed July 10, 2020, https://www.scienceofpeople.com/beauty-standards/.

3. Jonathan Vespa, Lauren Medina, and David M. Armstrong, *Demographic Turning Points* for the United States: *Population Projections for 2020 to 2060* (United States Census Bureau, Issued March 2018 and Revised February 2020), https://www.census.gov/content/dam/Census/library/publications/2020/demo/p25-1144.pdf.

4. "Older People Projected to Outnumber Children for First Time in U.S. History," United States Census Bureau, released March 13, 2018, revised September 6, 2018 and October 8, 2019, https://www.census.gov/newsroom/press-releases/2018/cb18-41-population-projections.html.

5. "Wellness Industry Statistics & Facts," Global Wellness Institute, October 2018, https://globalwellnessinstitute.org/press-room/statistics-and-facts/.

6. "List of Diets," *Wikipedia*, accessed June 3, 2021, https://wikipedia.org/wiki/List_of_diets.

Chapter 2: Your Body Works for You

1. *Merriam-Webster*, s.v. "calling (*n.*)," accessed August 1, 2021, https://www.merriam-webster.com/dictionary/calling.

Chapter 3: Do Unto Others. Period.

1. Susan Reynolds, "Happy Brain, Happy Life," *Psychology Today*, posted August 2, 2011, https://www.psychologytoday.com/us/blog/prime-your-gray-cells/201108/happy-brain-happy-life.

2. "The Power of Positive Thinking," Johns Hopkins Medicine, accessed April 23, 2021, https://www.hopkinsmedicine.org/health/wellness-and-prevention/the-power-of-positive-thinking.

3. Tara L. Kraft and Sarah D. Pressman, "Grin and Bear It: The Influence of Manipulated Facial Expression on the Stress Response," *Psychological Science* 23, no. 11 (published September 24, 2012), https://pubmed.ncbi.nlm.nih.gov/23012270/.

4. Daniel Muscat, "Positivity Matters: How Positive Thinking and Emotions Influence Physical Health and Well-Being" (bachelor's dissertation, L-Universitá ta' Malta, 2019), https://www.um.edu.mt/library/oar/handle/123456789/56601.

5. Arianna Huffington, "Evicting the Obnoxious Roommate in Your Head," Thrive Global, *Medium*, November 30, 2016, https://medium.com/thrive-global/evicting-the-obnoxious-roommate-in-your-head-1848db7c9d75.

6. Sanjay Gupta, *Keep Sharp* (New York: Simon & Schuster, 2021), 89.

7. Giuseppa Piras et al., "Immuno-moodulin: A New Anxiogenic Factor Produced by Annexin-A1 Transgenic Autoimmune-Prone T Cells," *Brain, Behavior, and Immunity* 87 (July 2020), https://www.sciencedirect.com/science/article/abs/pii/S0889159119315600.

8. Natalie L. Merchant et al., "Repetitive negative thinking is associated with amyloid, tau, and cognitive decline," Alzheimer's & Dementia, June 2, 2020, https://alz-journals.onlinelibrary.wiley.com/doi/10.1002/alz.12116.

9. "Worries on Your Mind," *Harvard Health*, October 1, 2020, https://www.health.harvard.edu/mind-and-mood/worries-on-your-mind.

10. Elizabeth Barbour, *Smart Self-Care for Busy Women* (2020), chap. 1., Kindle.

11. Saundra Dalton-Smith, *Sacred Rest* (New York: FaithWords, 2017), 127.

12. Sanjay Gupta, *Keep Sharp* (New York: Simon & Schuster, 2021), 149.

13. Sanjay Gupta, *Keep Sharp* (New York: Simon & Schuster, 2021), 149.

14. Matthew Thorpe and Rachael Link, "12 Science-Based Benefits of Meditation," Healthline, updated October 27, 2020, accessed April 2021, https://www.healthline.com/nutrition/12-benefits-of-meditation.

15. Ayman Mukerji Househam et al., "The Effects of Stress and Meditation on the Immune System, Human Microbiota, and Epigenetics," *Advances in Mind-Body Medicine* 31, no. 4 (Fall 2017), https://pubmed.ncbi.nlm.nih.gov/29306937/.

16. Jennie Allen, *Get Out of Your Head* (Colorado Springs: WaterBrook, 2020).

17. Bessel van der Kolk, *The Body Keeps the Score* (New York: Penguin Books, 2014), 81.

18. Bessel van der Kolk, The Body Keeps the Score (New York: Penguin Books, 2014).

Chapter 4: She Has THE Perfect Body

1. Malini Ghoshal, "What You Need to Know About Set Point Theory," Healthline, March 19, 2020, accessed March 2021, https://www.healthline.com/health/set-point-theory.html.

2. Billy Hawkins, Raegan A. Tuff, and Gary Dudley, "African American Women, Body Composition, and Physical Activity," *Journal of African American Studies* 10 (2006), https://doi.org/10.1007/s12111-006-1012-5.

3. "The System Is Failing Latinas and Black Women," *Lean In*, accessed March 2021, https://leanin.org/research/equal-pay-day-2021#!

4. Adele Jackson-Gibson, "The Racist and Problematic History of the Body Mass Index," *Good Housekeeping*, February 23, 2021, https://www.goodhousekeeping.com/health/diet-nutrition/a35047103/bmi-racist-history.

5. Sabrina Strings, *Fearing the Black Body* (New York: New York University Press, 2019), 9.

6. Adele Jackson-Gibson, "The Racist and Problematic History of the Body Mass Index," *Good Housekeeping*, February 23, 2021, https://www.goodhousekeeping.com/health/diet-nutrition/a35047103/bmi-racist-history.

Chapter 5: I Can Tell You're Healthy by Looking at You

1. *Merriam-Webster*, s.v. "weight (n.)," accessed August 1, 2021, http://www.merriam-webster.com/dictionary/weight.

2. World Health Organization, *Waist Circumference and Waist-Hip Ratio: Report of a WHO Expert Consultation* (World Health Organization, 2011), https://www.who.int/publications/i/item/9789241501491.

3. American Heart Association News, "Waist Size Predicts Heart Attacks Better Than BMI, Especially in Women," American Heart Association, February 28, 2018, https://www.heart.org/en/news/2019/03/19/waist-size-predicts-heart-attacks-better-than-bmi-especially-in-women.

4. Cuilin Zhang et al., "Abdominal Obesity and the Risk of All-Cause, Cardiovascular, and Cancer Mortality: Sixteen Years of Follow-Up in US Women," *Circulation* 117, no. 13 (April 1, 2008), https://pubmed.ncbi.nlm.nih.gov/18362231/.

5. JP Després, "Health Consequences of Visceral Obesity," *Annals of Medicine* 33, no. 8 (November 2001), https://pubmed.ncbi.nlm.nih.gov/11730160/.

6. Goran Medic, Micheline Wille, and Michiel EH Hemels, "Short- and Long-Term Health Consequences of Sleep Disruption," *Nature and Science of Sleep* 9 (May 19, 2017), https://www.ncbi.nlm.nih.gov/pmc/articles/PMC5449130/.

7. Nathaniel F. Watson et al., "Recommended Amount of Sleep for a Healthy Adult: A Joint Consensus Statement of the American Academy of Sleep Medicine and Sleep Research Society," *Sleep Research Society* 38, no. 6 (June 1, 2015), https://www.ncbi.nlm.nih.gov/pmc/articles/PMC4434546/.

8. Sanjay Gupta, *Keep Sharp* (New York: Simon & Schuster, 2021), 138.

9. Goran Medic, Micheline Wille, and Michiel EH Hemels, "Short- and Long-Term Health Consequences of Sleep Disruption," *Nature and Science of Sleep* 9 (May 19, 2017), https://www.ncbi.nlm.nih.gov/pmc/articles/PMC5449130/.

10. "Stress Effects on the Body," American Psychological Association, November 1, 2018, https://www.apa.org/topics/stress/body.

11. "10 Ways Sleep Deprivation Affects Your Health," Cleveland Clinic, August 23, 2019, https://health.clevelandclinic.org/10-ways-sleep-deprivation-affects-your-health/.

12. Eric Suni, "Healthy Sleep Tips," Sleep Foundation, July 30, 2020, https://www.sleepfoundation.org/sleep-hygiene/healthy-sleep-tips.

13. Sanjay Gupta, *Keep Sharp* (New York: Simon & Schuster, 2021), 132.

14. Sanjay Gupta, *Keep Sharp* (New York: Simon & Schuster, 2021), 107.

15. Leonardo Barbosa Barreto de Brito et al., "Ability to Sit and Rise from the Floor as a Predictor of All-Cause Mortality," *European Journal of Preventive Cardiology* (2012), https://geriatrictoolkit.missouri.edu/srff/deBrito-Floor-Rise-Mortality-2012.pdf.

16. American Heart Association Editorial Staff, "Understanding Blood Pressure Readings," American Heart Association, accessed October 6, 2021, https://www.heart.org/en/health-topics/high-blood-pressure/understanding-blood-pressure-readings.

Chapter 6: I Have to Work Off Dessert

1. Caroline Leaf, *Think and Eat Yourself Smart* (Grand Rapids: Baker Publishing Group, 2016), 84.

Chapter 7: It's All About the Nutrients

1. Shauna Niequist, Bread and Wine (Grand Rapids: Zondervan, 2013), https://www.amazon.com/Bread-Wine-Letter-Around-Recipes-ebook/dp/B008EGV68M/ref=sr_1_1?crid=1E3ALGJA56GGE&dchild =1&keywords=bread+and+wine+shauna+niequist&qid=1626455073& sprefix=bread+and+wine%2Caps%2C618&sr=8-1.

2. Dictionary.com, s.v. "nourish (*v.*)," accessed August 1, 2021, https://www.dictionary.com/browse/nourish.

Chapter 8: Carbs are the Enemy

1. American Heart Association Editorial Staff, "Added Sugars," American Heart Association, April 17, 2018, https://www.heart.org/en/healthy-living/healthy-eating/eat-smart/sugar/added-sugars.

2. F Erbsloh, A Bernsmeier, and H Hillesheim, "The Glucose Consumption of the Brain and Its Dependence on the Liver," *Arch Psychiatr Nervenkr Z Gesamte Neurol Psychiatr* 196, no. 6 (1958), https://pubmed.ncbi.nlm.nih.gov/13534602/.

3. E.C. LaMeaux, "How to Calculate Your Ideal Body Fat Percentage," Gaiam, accessed November 2020, https://www.gaiam.com/blogs/discover/how-to-calculate-your-ideal-body-fat-percentage.

4. Kristin W. Barañano and Adam L. Hartman, "The Ketogenic Diet: Uses in Epilepsy and other Neurologic Illnesses," *Current Treatment Options in Neurology* 10, no. 6 (November 2008), https://www.ncbi.nlm.nih.gov/pmc/articles/PMC2898565/.

5. "Ketogenic Diets," National Academy of Sports Medicine Nutrition Certification, accessed June 2020.

Chapter 9: There's One Best Diet

1. "Dietary Reference Intakes for Macronutrients," The National Academies of Sciences Engineering Medicine, 2005, https://www. nationalacademies.org/our-work/dietary-reference-intakes-for-macronutrients.

2. Evelyn Tribole, "What Is Intuitive Eating?" Intuitive Eating, September 12, 2018, https://www.intuitiveeating.org/what-is-intuitive-eating-tribole/.

Chapter 10: Jump In and Get 'Er Done

1. Sarah M. Marek et al., "Acute Effects of Static and Proprioceptive Neuromuscular Facilitation Stretching on Muscle Strength and Power Output," *Journal of Athletic Training* 40, no. 2 (April–June 2005), https://www.ncbi.nlm.nih.gov/pmc/articles/PMC1150232/.

Chapter 12: Working Out Is Too Complicated

1. Pete McCall, "Functional Anatomy Series: The Shoulders," ACE Fitness, July 2016, https://www.acefitness.org/education-and-resources/professional/prosource/july-2016/5978/functional-anatomy-series-the-shoulders/.

Chapter 13: I Don't Want to Bulk Up by Strength Training

1. J.C. Aristizabal et al., "Effect of Resistance Training on Resting Metabolic Rate and Its Estimation by a Dual-Energy X-ray Absorptiometry Metabolic Map," *European Journal of Clinical Nutrition* 69, no. 7 (October 8, 2014), https://pubmed.ncbi.nlm.nih.gov/25293431/.

2. Harri Suominen, "Muscle Training for Bone Strength," *Aging Clinical and Experimental Research* 18, no. 2 (April 2006), https://pubmed.ncbi.nlm.nih.gov/16702776/.

3. Darren T. Beck et al., "Exercise Training Improves Endothelial Function in Young Prehypertensives," *Experimental Biology and Medicine* (Maywood, N.J.) 238, no. 4 (April 2013), https://pubmed.ncbi.nlm.nih.gov/23760009/.

4. Zachary Mang et al., "Metabolic Effects of Resistance Training," Len Kravitz/The University of New Mexico, accessed October 2020, https://www.unm.edu/~lkravitz/Article%20folder/metaboliceffectsofRT.html.

5. Zachary Mang et al., "Metabolic Effects of Resistance Training," Len Kravitz/The University of New Mexico, accessed October 2020, https://www.unm.edu/~lkravitz/Article%20folder/metaboliceffectsofRT.html.

Chapter 14: I Have to Get My Hour of Exercise In

1. U.S. Department of Health and Human Services, 2008 *Physical Activity Guidelines for Americans*, 2008, https://health.gov/sites/default/files/2019-09/paguide.pdf.

2. Ulf Ekelund et al., "Joint Associations of Accelerometer-Measured Physical Activity and Sedentary Time with All-Cause Mortality: A Harmonised Meta-analysis in More Than 44 000 Middle-Aged and Older Individuals," *British Journal of Sports Medicine* 54, no. 24 (December 2020), https://bjsm.bmj.com/content/54/24/1499.

3. Len Kravitz, *HIIT Your Limit* (Apollo Publishers, 2018), 26-30.

4. Len Kravitz, *HIIT Your Limit* (Apollo Publishers, 2018), 22.

5. Pete McCall, "Exercise and Hormones: 8 Hormones Involved in Exercise," ACE Fitness, August 10, 2015, https://www.acefitness.org/education-and-resources/professional/expert-articles/5593/exercise-and-hormones-8-hormones-involved-in-exercise/.

6. Len Kravitz, "A NEAT 'New' Strategy for Weight Control," Len Kravitz/The University of New Mexico, accessed September 2020, https://www.unm.edu/~lkravitz/Article%20folder/NeatLK.html.

7. Len Kravitz, "New Clues to Prevent Weight Regain," Len Kravitz/The University of New Mexico, accessed September 2020, https://www.unm.edu/~lkravitz/Article%20folder/WeightRegain.html.

8. Charles E. Matthews et al., "Mortality Benefits for Replacing Sitting Time with Different Physical Activities," *Medicine and Science in Sports and Exercise* 47, no. 9 (September 2015), https://pubmed.ncbi.nlm.nih.gov/25628179/.

9. Len Kravitz, "Move 3 for Every 30," Len Kravitz/The University of New Mexico, 2018, https://www.unm.edu/~lkravitz/Article%20folder/move3forevery30.html.

10. Pete McCall, "6 Things to Know About Non-exercise Activity Thermogenesis," *ACE Fitness, November 21, 2017, https://www. acefitness.org/education-and-resources/lifestyle/blog/6852/6-things-to-know-about-non-exercise-activity-thermogenesis/.*

Chapter 15: No Pain, No Gain

1. *Merriam-Webster*, s.v. "pain (*n.*)," accessed August 1, 2021, https://www.merriam-webster.com/dictionary/pain.

2. *Merriam-Webster*, s.v. "health (*n.*)," accessed August 1, 2021, https://www.merriam-webster.com/dictionary/health.

Chapter 16: Pass the Bucket

1. Pawel Samborski, Anna Chmielarz-Czarnocińska, and Marian Grzymisławski, "Exercise-Induced Vomiting," *Przegląd Gastroenterologiczny Gastroenterology Review* 8, no. 6 (2013), https://www.ncbi.nlm.nih.gov/pmc/articles/PMC4027831/.

2. Sarah Schlichter, "The Top 5 Reasons Why You Experience Nausea After Running," *Women's Running*, July 28, 2021, https://www.womensrunning.com/health/post-workout-nauseous-stomach-upset/.

3. Shawn H. Dolan, "Electrolytes: Understanding Replacement Options," ACE Fitness, accessed September 2020, https://www.acefitness.org/certifiednewsarticle/715/electrolytes-understanding-replacement-options/.

4. Isha Shrimanker and Sandeep Bhattarai, "Electrolytes," in *StatPearls* (Treasure Island, FL: StatPearls Publishing), https://www.ncbi.nlm.ih.gov/books/NBK541123/.

5. United States Department of Agriculture, *Scientific Report of the 2015 Dietary Guidelines Advisory Committee*, 2015, https://health.gov/sites/default/files/2019-09/Scientific-Report-of-the-2015-Dietary-Guidelines-Advisory-Committee.pdf.

Chapter 17: Walking Isn't a Real Workout

1. National Academy of Sports Medicine (NASM), *NASM Essentials of Personal Fitness Training*, 6th ed. (Burlington: Jones & Bartlett Learning, 2018), 226.

2. Pete McCall, *Smarter Workouts: The Science of Exercise Made Simple* (Champaign: Human Kinetics, 2019), 114.

3. Pete McCall, *Smarter Workouts: The Science of Exercise Made Simple* (Champaign: Human Kinetics, 2019), 289.

4. Kelly McGonigal, *The Joy of Movement* (New York: Avery Publishing, 2019), 18.

5. Kelly McGonigal, *The Joy of Movement* (New York: Avery Publishing, 2019), 53.

6. Kelly McGonigal, *The Joy of Movement*, (New York: Avery Publishing, 2019), 62.

7. Teresa Dumain, "Walking with Arthritis: Benefits, Tips, How to Prevent Pain," CreakyJoints, November 15, 2019, https://creakyjoints.org/diet-exercise/walking-with-arthritis/.

8. Apichai Wattanapisit and Sanhapan Thanamee, "Evidence Behind 10,000 Steps Walking," *Journal of Health Research and Reviews in Developing Countries* 31, no. 3 (June 2017), https://www.thaiscience.info/journals/Article/JHRE/10985252.pdf.

9. "2011 Compendium of Physical Activities," https://cdn-links.lww.com/permalink/mss/a/mss_43_8_2011_06_13_ainsworth_202093_sdc1.pdf.

Chapter 18: There's One Right Way to Exercise

1. *Merriam-Webster*, s.v. "fetishize (*v.*)," accessed August 1, 2021, https://www.merriam-webster.com/dictionary/fetishize.

2. *Merriam-Webster*, s.v. "fetish (*n.*)," accessed August 1, 2021, https://www.merriam-webster.com/dictionary/fetish.

3. National Academy of Sports Medicine (NASM), NASM *Essentials of Personal Fitness Training*, 6th ed. (Burlington: Jones & Bartlett Learning, 2018), 367.

4. Pete McCall, *Smarter Workouts: The Science of Exercise Made Simple* (Champaign: Human Kinetics, 2019), 278.

Chapter 19: To Lose Weight, I Need to Exercise More and Eat Less

1. Jade Teta, *Metabolic Renewal Road Map* (Metabolic Living), 4..

2. National Academy of Sports Medicine (NASM), *NASM Essentials of Personal Fitness Training*, 6th ed. (Burlington: Jones & Bartlett Learning, 2018), 215.

3. Jade Teta, M*etabolic Renewal Road Map* (Metabolic Living), 4.

4. Jade Teta, *Metabolic Renewal Road Map* (Metabolic Living), 4.

Chapter 20: No Rest for the Weary

1. Pete McCall, "8 Reasons to Take a Rest Day," ACE Fitness, December 19, 2018, https://www.acefitness.org/education-and-resources/lifestyle/blog/7176/8-reasons-to-take-a-rest-day/.

2. Pete McCall, "8 Reasons to Take a Rest Day," ACE Fitness, December 19, 2018, https://www.acefitness.org/education-and-resources/lifestyle/blog/7176/8-reasons-to-take-a-rest-day/.

3. Scott W. Cheatham et al., "The Effects of Self-Myofascial Release Using a Foam Roll or Roller Massager on Joint Range of Motion, Muscle Recovery, and Performance: A Systematic Review," *International Journal of Sports Physical Therapy* 10, no. 6 (November 2015), https://www.ncbi.nlm.nih.gov/pmc/articles/PMC4637917/.

Chapter 21: It's a Waste of Time if I Don't Lose Weight

1. Glen Davison, Corinna Kehaya, and Arwel Wyn Jones, "Nutritional and Physical Activity Interventions to Improve Immunity," *American Journal of Lifestyle Medicine* 10, no. 3 (May–June 2016), https://www.ncbi.nlm.nih.gov/pmc/articles/PMC6124954/.

2. Kelly McGonigal, *The Joy of Movement* (New York: Avery Publishing, 2019), 62.

3. Kelly McGonigal, *The Joy of Movement* (New York: Avery Publishing, 2019), 42.

4. Merriam-Webster, s.v. "weight (n.)," accessed August 1, 2021, https://www.merriam-webster.com/dictionary/weight.

Made in the USA
Columbia, SC
12 November 2021